Starting a Chiropractic Practice

a comprehensive guide to clinic management

Starting a Chiropractic Practice

a comprehensive guide to clinic management

Gayle A. Jensen
Rudolf P. Vrugtman

Foreword by
George A. Goodman
President, Logan College of Chiropractic
and
Elizabeth A. Parrott
Vice Chair, Board of Trustees, Logan College of Chiropractic

Rudi Publishing
San Francisco

Rudi Publishing, 12 Geary St. #508, San Francisco, CA 94108

First Edition 1990
Second Edition 1992
Third Edition 1997

ISBN 0-945213-25-5

Printed in the United States of America by Vaughan Printing

Library of Congress Cataloging-in-Publication Data

Jensen, Gayle A.,
    Starting a chiropractic practice : a comprehensive guide to
clinic management / Gayle A. Jensen, Rudolf P. Vrugtman ; foreword
by George A. Goodman and Elizabeth A. Parrott. — [Rev. 3rd ed.]
    p.   cm.
    Includes bibliographical references and index.
    ISBN 0-945213-25-5
    1. Chiropractic—Practice.   I. Vrugtman, Rudolf P.
II. Title.
    [DNLM: 1. Chiropractic—organization & administration. 2.
Private Practice—organization & administration. 3. Professional
Practice--organization & administration.   WB 905.7 J54s 1997]
RZ232.2.J46 1997
615.5'34'068—dc21
DNLM/DLC
for Library of Congress   97-18284
    CIP

In business, the earning of profit is something more than an incident of success. It is an essential condition of success. It is an essential condition of success because the continued absence of profit itself spells failure.

Justice Louis D. Brandeis

*If one advances confidently in the direction of his dreams,
and endeavors to live the life which he has imagined,
he will meet with a success unexpected in common hours.*

Henry David Thoreau

*Six essential qualities that are the key to success:
Sincerity, personal integrity, humility, courtesy, wisdom, charity.*

Dr. William Menninger

Contents

Foreword

The Ethical Landscape

Ms. Gayle Jensen and Mr. Rudi Vrugtman have provided a significant contribution to chiropractic education. Their efforts to provide information that will increase the business acumen of the individual studying chiropractic and of the seasoned chiropractic physician are essential to chiropractic education. In addition, they provide a tremendous source of information. It is expected that chiropractic health-care providers, as educated men and women, acquire a significant level of informed judgment. This informed judgment enables the student and practitioner to be prepared to make discriminating moral choices. We applaud Ms. Jensen and Mr. Vrugtman for recognizing this need in chiropractic education.

The question of ethics is high on society's list of qualities and expectations in health-care providers as well as those of significant leadership positions in the public or private sector. The question of ethics in 1996 was revisited in the most recent presidential election through the antics of the Speaker of the House of Representatives, and even the military has dealt with its ethical and moral quality to train combat-ready personnel without harassment.

Borrowing from the game of golf, we find many golfers who divide the game into two components. The first section is the number of shots from tee to green. The second portion of the game is discussed as the number of putts from green to the cup. So it is in chiropractic practice.

We have the moral, legal, and ethical behavior, as well as duties and responsibilities to care for the patient on one hand, and on the other hand the secondary component of ethical, legal, and moral application of the same principles to the third-party payor. This could imply the government, insurance carriers, managed care organizations, or the documentation of patient SOAP notes as the secondary component. Keep in mind—the last time we checked, it was the duty and responsibility of the practitioner to complete venues with the same sense of moral and ethical obligation. Our example of golf indicated that every stroke from tee to cup will continue to count the same, unless the rules are changed. When you add up your score card, or address patient results in case management, the winner will be the player or practitioner who counted every stroke and addressed every component of practice, in regulation. (H. Penick, *The Game for a Lifetime,* p. 81)

Individual Ethics

> The affectation of universities is the pretense that everyone is ethically sophisticated to start with, a striking example of self deception. Some companies and agencies offer formal codes of ethics, but reading code is like reading a regulation: unless the ideas and values are internalized, their written form is itself a form of deception.
>
> Robert Payton
> (T. Pezzullo and P. Brittingham,
> *Fund Raising in Higher Education: Ethical Questions,* p.3)

The above quotation is reminiscent of dilemmas that many of us find ourselves in when we attempt to "fix the blame fast" when something goes awry. The dilemma of spending time on worrying about "who's right" rather than mentally deliberating and deciding "what's right" faces each of us in patient care giving. The need for a deliberate set of ethical values is the minimum requirement for a doctor of chiropractic to practice and perform service. The doctor who develops the tendency to cut the corner of societal and professional ethical and moral standards will be ultimately held accountable. The loss of trust as applied to the doctor/patient relationship along with loss of professional credibility marks the individual practitioner in a very negative context.

The doctor of chiropractic who took advantage of his/her patient by not conforming to a standard of "what is right," or who developed a relationship of sexual misconduct, established the rationale for the various layers of bureaucratic rules and practice regulations that have been developed by individual states. The "right" to practice chiropractic is based upon education and legislative practice acts. If the right is violated, it leads to the loss of the right to practice, or the loss of licensure. The *privilege* to practice chiropractic is based upon the legislated mandate which in most states requires proper patient protocols, diagnosis, treatment plans, and patient consent, in following the established ethical standards of the chiropractic profession, as expected and demanded by the health-seeking consumer. The ethical components that relate to our patient relationships must always continue in our business practice and procedures.

Both doctors of chiropractic and chiropractic students, by virtue of their academic education and their position in the community as professionals, represent the chiropractic profession as a whole. They therefore have a duty to exemplify the best qualities of the institution they are or have been associated with, and the communities they currently work within. The highest standards of personal and professional conduct are expected of professionals in all arenas of their expertise. All organizations—institutional, state-mandated, and professional—supply codes of ethics for the guidance of the professional reputation of the doctor of chiropractic. Within each of these codes are guidelines that seek to promote the merit of the chiropractic profession without disparaging other health-care professions. Ethics embodies a respect for truth, fairness, and the opinions of others, without regard to race, creed, color, sexual orientation, ethnicity, or impairments. Privacy, confidentiality, and the avoidance of conflicts of interest are the foundational principles upon which the individual ethics of the doctor of chiropractic are based. The growth of the chiropractic profession, its complexity, and sophistication have resulted in ethical issues associated with lifestyles, complex patient relationships, and third-party payors that didn't exist a decade ago.

Ethics Beyond the Individual

The chiropractic profession has historically seen multiplicities of business ventures in the areas of practice management. Far too often, and admittedly embarrassingly, the "hot" group or organizational techniques provided a greed factor which has been detrimental to our professional growth and development. The new millennium standards will be based on sound ethical business skills taught to the chiropractic student and held by seasoned practitioners. These new skills will be part of the educational partnerships that will combine them with technical skills, procedures, business protocols, and marketing—partnerships that integrate efforts from the universities' schools of business and the chiropractic educational community.

The new millennium provides great hope and exciting challenge for the expansion of educational partnerships which will continually foster and develop trust between the doctor of chiropractic and the potential chiropractic patient. As our consortium of chiropractic colleges develop the needed and necessary higher educational partnerships, the academic cross training will foster a greater degree of confidence, not only in the public's mind, but in the treating practitioner's mind. The principle of chiropractic itself is as ethically and morally right as any health-care profession in existence. Its practitioners represent a nonsurgical, drugless, conservative health-care delivery system.

The ethical behavior of the doctor of chiropractic can fit easily into the analogy of a high handicapper playing golf on a course designed to force the golfer into playing an uncomfortably difficult game. The course the golfer plays, and the tee the golfer chooses to fit his or her ability, are the same choices the chiropractor faces in choosing the method of practice and the proper behavior necessary in practice. The course must fit the game the golfer knows how to play. Ethical practice must fit the education and standards the chiropractor has acquired. (Penick, p. 60-61)

The doctor of chiropractic has developed levels of professional competency and informed acquaintance. This professional competence and informed acquaintance is the area that the practitioner has "majored in" and has provided mental "concentration." This cumulative learning has provided us with the development of powers of reasoning and analysis including analytical constructs. (H. Rosofsky, *The University: An Owner's Manual*, p. 107)

It is expected, therefore, that the student, and, ultimately, the clinician has gained sufficient control of the ability to document patient data and methods to define and differentiate the clinical issues that patients present. The outcome and evidence to treat the patient effectively is assumed. Society expects a "reasonable" standard of ethical and clinical behavior as the first level of clinical competence.

There is a vast difference between a moral foundation and a legal situation. Yet the two seem to relate to individual values and a set of values that the doctor chooses as principles to live by. In the case of loss of moral foundation, accountability becomes the factor. A moral infraction relates to a loss of trust, credibility, and, ultimately, patients. Whereas, legal accountability can cause everything from the feared audit to a loss of licensure or the right to practice the profession. Morality is a public system that applies to all moral agents or persons who are held responsible for their actions. Individuals are subject to morality simply by virtue of being rational and by combining this with sufficient knowledge and values to be held responsible for their actions. It is necessary to understand what it means to act in an ethical and moral landscape (D. Elliott, *Ethics of Asking: Dilemma in Higher Education Fundraising*, pp. 30-32). It permits actions combined with special role-related responsibilities that totally relate to what an individual should or should not be involved in.

Experience has shown us that the doctor of chiropractic should be assertive and strong. Of prime importance is the fundamental behavior that comes from morality, sincerity, decency, respect for others, personal goodness, and true caring. These humanistic characteristics must shine through in a professional's behavior, as no application of practice management procedures or style will work without the above characteristics. The doctor of chiropractic must maintain a fidelity in his or her relationships with all individuals. Probably one of the best testing devices is to wake up each morning, look in the bathroom mirror, and ask whether or not what one does is in the best interest of the patients one serves—one patient at a time. Today, effective doctors of chiropractic are characterized by a strong drive for responsibility, the appearance of vigor, persistence, a willingness to take chances, originality, a sense of humor, social initiative, self confidence, decisiveness, a sense of identity, personal style, a capacity to organize, a predisposition to action, and a willingness to absorb the stress of others. In summary, the effective and ethical practitioner must have a desire for impact and for being strong and influential, set in an arena that is greater than the desire for personal achievement (J. Fisher, *Power of the Presidency*).

The following observations (H. Brown, *Life's Little Instruction Book*, pp. 16, 33, 211, 218, 234, 241) represent thoughts to guide an individual through the ethical landscape:

- Respect tradition
- Teach your children the value of money and the importance of saving.
- Commit yourself to constant self improvement
- Take your dog to obedience school. You'll both learn a lot.
- Be the first to say "hello."
- Treat everyone you meet like you want to be treated.
- Cultivate patients and keep the common touch. (George Goodman)

George A. Goodman, D.C., F.I.C.C.
President, Logan College of Chiropractic

Elizabeth A. Parrott, D.C.
Vice Chair, Board of Trustees
Logan College of Chiropractic

Preface to the Third, Revised Edition

We have changed and so has the world around us. The chiropractic profession has not stood still since we first published this book in 1990. There has been change all around us, we have received further formal education, and we have been exposed to many more chiropractors—the good and the not so good. We have become more involved in the profession and our love for it and its place in our society has grown.

Our students have given us the honor of listening to us and of trying to implement some of our ideas and concepts. Most who really tried have succeeded because of the energy and effort they invested, yet some insist on doing us the honor of crediting us with their success.

Chiropractic is a business. Yes, chiropractors try to help other people live a better life, but without business and financial survival, such attempts have to end. The population is becoming more open to what it calls alternative health care. In the process, people are beginning to recognize that waiting for the breakdown of the body, when drastic measures such as drugs and surgery may be the only realistic alternative, is not the route leading to good health. Chiropractors, with their holistic and preventative attitude toward health, are therefore primed to be the growth profession in the health-care industry in most countries. We are convinced that the new generation of chiropractors is ready to accept that challenge. We are convinced, as well, that this generation will perform superbly.

As will be obvious to the reader of prior editions, we have completely revised and updated this edition. Some of this reflects the growth of the authors over the last seven years, some of it is necessitated by changes in the profession. Most exciting of all are those changes caused by the improvements in chiropractic education. We feel certain that you, the reader and user of this book, will have suggestions for us to improve and add in future editions. Please do not hesitate to send us your comments. Some people complain about the rapid change in technology, but we love it. Communication today is much easier and quicker than only a few years ago. Both of us are on line and will gladly receive your e-mail. Time permitting, we will try to respond.

Our wish is that this effort may assist you in making a better life for yourself, your family, but most of all, your patients.

Gayle A. Jensen   Rudolf P. Vrugtman
North Liberty, Iowa   Ballwin, Missouri

February 1997

Preface to the Second Edition

When, in the summer of 1990, we were finalizing this creation, we knew this work was needed in the chiropractic community. We had no idea how it would fare. Never in our wildest dreams did we anticipate the wholehearted acceptance that resulted.

The chiropractic education institutions, and the profession as a whole, have been extremely kind and complimentary. Our book is now used as a recommended or required text in six chiropractic colleges: Cleveland (Los Angeles), Life (West), Logan, New York Chiropractic, Palmer, and Pennsylvania College of Straight Chiropractic. National, Northwestern, and Parker have honored us with orders, as have numerous individuals and clinics. Even some of the "practice management" firms have ordered copies.

We have been invited to seminars at two colleges and have had tremendous fun assisting students, faculty members, and field doctors with "aha" factors and new discoveries, while learning a few things ourselves. The ego income from all of this is indeed tremendous, and there is no way we can thank you adequately.

Most gratifying, however, is the fact that we have to do a second run on the printing. We have made no material changes in this, preferring to allow a good, well-received product to continue. Minor changes have been made, some as a result of law changes.

It is the intent of the authors, the next time around, to revise and expand as required. If, in reading, using, or otherwise marking up this book, you would like us to address or expand certain areas, please feel free to let us know. We want this to be an up-to-date, useful tool for new chiropractors coming into the profession. In the back of this book you will find a tear-out page for your comments. We hope you use it.

Finally, let us assure you that our purpose is to benefit the chiropractic profession. Education is the road every profession has taken to improve the product it supplies the consuming public. We hope to continue to be of assistance in the growth of the chiropractic profession, for the ultimate purpose of providing excellent health care to the world.

Gayle A. Jensen   Rudolf P. Vrugtman
North Liberty, Iowa   Ballwin, Missouri

Acknowledgments

The theories, thoughts, ideas, and systems expressed in this work are not original. Many individuals and texts have been used as sources of knowledge over the last twenty years by the authors in their business and management positions. Where appropriate, direct quotations and sources have been recognized and acknowledged. It is impossible to trace all ideas, theories, and expressions to their original innovators. Instead of attempting such activity, the authors hereby recognize the tremendous support received from all those who have gone before.

A work of this nature, once its desirability becomes obvious, is the full responsibility of the authors who undertake its creation. As the song says, though, " ... with a little help from my friends" everything becomes easier. In this endeavor there have been many friends, not all of whom can be named. We trust they know who they are, and that we appreciate their help and support. They have spent nearly two decades teaching us to think, to observe, and to strive for excellence. We hope we deliver.

A few specific thanks are in order to

Kevin Bays, D.C., for being an accepting student who proves us right

Benjamin Blackstock, J.D., for belief and guidance

Terri Boekhoff, for striving for excellence

Charles Bratkowski, C.P.S., for contributions and rough drafts for the first edition

Richard Cranwell, D.C., for support, encouragement, and an introduction to chiropractic

William Davis, for being himself

George Goodman, D.C., for being a friend and for wishing the best for his profession

Gary Johnson, D.C., for continuous encouragement and his desire for the best possible

Richard Koelling, D.C., for sketches and observations

Tom Kriz, for thoughts, friendship, and trust

Carl Lothman, J.D., for brain power and understanding

Irwin Neufeld, D.C., for succor and openness

Elizabeth Parrot, D.C., for insight and understanding

David Swope, D.C., for opening one author's world to chiropractic, for reassurance, and advice

Our families for all of the attributes above, but especially for patience and tolerance.

Above all, it needs to be clear that every word in this text is the sole responsibility of the authors.

Part One

So You Want To Be a Chiropractor

1

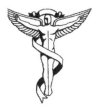 **Welcome to Entrepreneurship**

So you want to be a chiropractor. You came to school and decided to spend many years getting ready for something that you may, or may not, know much about. Some prospective students do know because there is a chiropractor in the family, some may have been in a chiropractor's office, and some have no idea. Maybe a counselor at your college told you chiropractors make pretty good money. What the prospective students did not see or realize, what the counselor did not say, is that chiropractors are also business owners. In the United States of America, Canada, and Europe, most chiropractors at some time during their career own their own practice. You will be a small business owner, an entrepreneur.

Maybe you are a practicing chiropractor and picked up the book because you are not running the practice with the results you had envisioned when you started. Or, maybe you have been someone's employee (associate) and now want to prepare to start your own practice. Whatever the reason for reading this, congratulations! You have decided to learn a few things about running a practice. We, the authors, feel that what follows will help you whether you are a novice or a seasoned practitioner. We expect that you will find some thoughts, approaches, or procedures that will be helpful in developing your professional management skills. We hope that you will use whatever you find for the betterment of yourself, your practice, and the profession. But above all, we hope you will use it for the benefit of the ones who really count: the patients.

In their book, *Entrepreneurship, a Contemporary Approach,* Donald Kuratko and Richard Hodgett list and debunk (pp. 7–9) ten myths of entrepreneurship:

1. Entrepreneurs are doers, not thinkers.
2. Entrepreneurs are born, not made.
3. Entrepreneurs are either inventors or innovators.
4. Entrepreneurs are academic or social misfits.
5. Entrepreneurs must fit the "profile."
6. All you need is money to be an entrepreneur.
7. All you need is luck to be an entrepreneur.
8. Ignorance is bliss for an entrepreneur.
9. Entrepreneurs strike success on their first venture.
10. Five years marks the failure of most new ventures.

Clearly, as chiropractors are also entrepreneurs, a recognition of the fallacy of the myths must be present. The myths came about because there have been examples in which a single factor of success for a business appeared obvious to all observers. Reality shows, however, that entrepreneurs are doers and thinkers, that they have learned their skills and understandings, that they have short bursts of innovation and long drawn-out periods of humdrum effort, and so forth.

Being an entrepreneur, a practice owner, is hard work. It necessitates total immersion, especially in the beginning. It is constant learning, as a successful practice requires different management skills from the owner at the various stages of its life cycle. "Forming, storming, norming, and conforming" are periods in a business life that require adjustments in management style and in resources brought to bear on the issues of the period.

We would like you to realize that by becoming a chiropractor and entrepreneur you have chosen to accept risk as part of your life. Most of us define risk as uncertainty about the future. It has various facets—financial risk, for instance. When starting a business, *financial risk* is attached. The entrepreneur does not know what the income or cash flow will be. There is no certainty about the amount left over, or whether it will be adequate to live on. There is financial risk involved in coming to school. It is not cheap to get a professional education, and most students borrow money to pay the tuition and to live on during the period of schooling.

Some have accepted *career risk*. If you were previously in a quite good job, you may have been climbing the professional ladder in that position. You could have continued, you could have made it to the top—but you chose to walk away from that possibility, just because you had this internal drive, or this idea, or this dream. And now the former career opportunity is gone and there is only uncertainty about a career as a chiropractor.

Many have accepted *family risk*. Some students are going through this education and training process without the benefit of spouse or family, which may still be the old home town. The intent is to go back there upon graduation, meanwhile surviving a commuting marriage. The statistics of how entrepreneurs fare in their family environment are horrendous. The number of divorces in any professional school, including chiropractic school, and in the entrepreneurial period thereafter, are well beyond national norms.

Having accepted those risks, you will discover that there is another one that automatically shows up. Prepare to be willing to live with uncertainty, to accept financial, career, or family risk, which in turn lead to *psychic risk*. Let's face it—some people just are not cut out to live with uncertainty, and yet professionals are in a risk environment.

Reasons for Business Failure

All of us hear the scary statistics of how many new business ventures, and thus startup chiropractic offices, fail. Donald Kuratko and Richard Hodgett report on some studies done to determine the reasons for business failure. From this list (Kuratko and Hodgett, pp. 173–7) we abstracted the following factors as commonly applying to professionals:

1. Inadequate market knowledge
2. Ineffective marketing and sales efforts
3. Inadequate awareness of competitive pressures
4. Undercapitalization, unforeseen operating expenses, excessive investment in fixed assets, and related financial difficulties
5. Unclear business definition
6. Assuming too much debt too early
7. Relationship troubles with money sources

It is interesting to note that the first cause of failure on the list is that the business owner has inadequate market knowledge. This leads to the questions: What do you know about the health-care market? What do you know about what your potential patients want? What do you know about bringing potential patients into your office? About dealing with those folks? Most chiropractors and students do not have a realistic view of the health-care market. They are treated for free by colleagues or family, they understand the value of life-long preventative care, and they know the symptomatic relief that can be obtained from an adjustment. Does the general population share this knowledge?

The number two failure cause is ineffective marketing and sales efforts. In health-care professions, this becomes exacerbated by the attitude, "I am a doctor, I don't have to sell." Yet every entrepreneur is selling, all day, all the time. Professionals may not think of it as selling, they may wish it were not necessary, but it is in today's marketplace. In Chapter 3 the sales and marketing process will be dealt with.

The surveys showed as the number three reason for failure an inadequate awareness of the competitive pressures. Most interpretations of "competitive pressures" are incorrect. Chiropractors think of the other chiropractor across the street as the competitor, while in reality, the competition is not the other chiropractor, but all health-care providers. Not just the allopath, but the naturopath, the homeopath, and others as well. The competitor is also the blue curtains the patient wants to buy for the living room, or the new TV, or the tuition for the child's schooling. The question to be asked is, How do we assist potential patients in motivating themselves to want to spend priority family dollars on health care? Individual practitioners will follow it with, How do I assure an appropriate portion of those dollars coming to my office?

It is interesting to realize that money and business management factors are relatively lower on the list. This indicates that marketing and selling are crucial factors for success in all of today's industries. Certainly health care is no exception—we only have to pay minimal attention to the daily news to realize the veracity of this. Therefore, human relations skills are crucial to the success of chiropractic offices.

The money issues on the list are ranked fourth, sixth, and seventh. The management issue is listed in the middle: unclear business definition. It really has a marketing impact also: How can you effectively communicate what you do and who you are, if you have not drawn clear delineations and distinctions for yourself? We see it in our students, and in young professionals, and even in well established professionals. Who are you, really? What is chiropractic? What do chiropractors do, why do they exist, what is their purpose?

In reviewing the list, it is striking that all entries have to do with either a lack of planning or a subsidiary lack of appropriate information. There is a moral here: To be successful as a chiropractor, owning your own practice, there is a need to go through a period of thought and data gathering. In other words, a business plan will need to be written.

Reasons for Business Success
If there are reasons for business failure, there are also factors for entrepreneurial success. While most professionals expect their particular technical or clinical skills, such as good adjuster, excellent clinician, fantastic diagnostician, to be high on the list, it appears from survey respondents those are not important factors. A survey of professionals (lawyer, architects, accountants, and doctors) compiled for a thesis paper by one of our students indicated the following order of importance as developed in a self appraisal interview series:

1. Personality
2. Location
3. Collection for services rendered
4. Market knowledge
5. Financial management
6. Planning
7. Enjoying the effort
8. Providing value-added services to clients or patients
9. Low overhead
10. Interpersonal skills
11. Presence of a referral base
12. Clinical/technical capability
13. Knowledgeable staff and assistants
14. Personal outlook: attitude

While the authors were surprised to find location listed so high on the professional success factor list, there are no other surprises. The research confirms what we have perceived over more than two decades of working with entrepreneurs and professionals. The reason the clinical or technical skills are so low on the list, we surmise, is the presumptive presence of those in a professional. The customer's rationale runs along these lines: "She went to school to become a professional; that takes a long time, and she must pass a (state, national, professional) board exam to demonstrate capability. Therefore, I can pay attention to the factors important to me—the regulators pay attention to the skills." We, on the inside of the professions, know that this is not always correct. As Dr. Parrott and Dr. Goodman indicated in the foreword, we have a responsibility to the consuming public that our professional house be kept in order.

Be Prepared

Taking a step back to review, we find a scary picture. Many chiropractors start their own businesses. Many start right out of school. They walk across the stage on graduation day, people are smiling and shaking the graduate's hand. At the end of the stage, just before the graduate steps down, a piece of paper is stuck in his or her hand, and the graduate feels great. Back at the seat, the graduate opens the piece of paper, thinking it is a diploma, and is astonished to realize it is an $80,000–100,000 bill, now due and payable. The graduate, following the faculty mentor's suggestions, has just decided to start a practice from scratch, as soon as possible. Folks, if you want to talk about stress, this has to be the ultimate: living with risks not previously encountered, burdened by financial debt, planning to add more financial debt, and living for an undetermined period of time totally immersed in a business startup venture, being certain and uncertain at the same time about the clinical skills. Did Chiro Brothers College really prepare that graduate well enough for the future?

In moments of mature, calm reflection it is recognized that a professional practice will have an initial period which the authors call the "Valley of Death." It is a period in which cash flow is negative, turns around, and eventually becomes positive. More will be explained about this in Chapter 16 on finance. Suffice it to state here that suppliers, the landlord, utilities, and others will be delighted to work with you. Their attitude will be, "I'll provide the service or product, but I want payment now, at time of delivery." And yet, in the beginning of practice there are very few patients, therefore few services, thus few collections. This culminates in an initial period of negative cash flow. It then becomes a question of figuring out how deep the valley will be and how long it will take to climb out on the far rim. Stress, stress, stress!

In the days following graduation, the new doctor will be so focused in attitude, so excited about starting practice, that a normal reaction is to be impatient when communicating with other people. This leads to other stressors: relationship problems. The attitude will soon degenerate into, "Nobody likes me, nobody communicates with me, nobody understands me." And, because there are people problems, another stressor arrives: loneliness. In addition, there is that final internal stressor, which eventually is going to be a success factor, but in the beginning is a stress factor: the burning desire to succeed, the need to achieve.

Recognition that these kinds of stress factors are going to be present will allow for development of ways of dealing with them. An important first step is to avoid the hermit syndrome. Recognize that as a human you have a need for others, no matter how busy you are. Take the time for those others, spend some human interaction time. Allow yourself to relax with others. Bounce some ideas off others. And realize, please, that if you do it right, you don't have to be alone in running your practice. You have a vision, why not share it? Why not get other people to help you, why not delegate? How do you find those other people? Networking. If you spend time with other people, if you talk to them about your vision, some of them are going to grab that vision and say, "That is neat. I want to help—how can I?" The moral of the story is, you need to communicate. Also, get a life. Find an interest other than your practice that you can get excited about, spend some time on it. Don't be too one sided.

Some readers may interpret the foregoing as negative. After all, we have stated reality, the things that can go wrong, and we have started to explain some of the reasons why they happen. But reality is not negative, it is positive. What sometimes makes life difficult are the factors that we were not aware of, that come at us unexpectedly, like the pro quarterback being blind-sided just as he is going to pass. If they know this is probable, during the week before a game, the coaches and players are going to set up a screen around the quarterback. They are going to have some blockers around him; he is going to have a nice pocket for pass protection. Similarly, if in starting your practice, you know what the real world is likely to send your way, you know the pass rushers are coming and where they are coming from, then you prepare to take care of them. You can plan on them coming and you can deal with them. It then becomes a question of executing the plan.

We have used the analogy of a professional football team here and some of you might find that inappropriate. We do not. After all, those players are professionals also, in fact we call them pros—short for professional. Maybe we need to take a moment and look at the definition of a pro.

Professionals are persons who are good at what they are doing, and they know why they are good at it. In more academic terminology, a professional is a conscious, competent individual. Most people start out in life, no matter what the profession or occupation, as amateurs. Being unaware, incompetent. In progressing from the amateur status to the pro status, there appear to be two routes possible. First, competency can be developed. Practice, practice, practice: set them up, do the adjustment, set them up, do the adjustment, do it right. After twenty, forty, a hundred times, you will get it right every time. Maybe it takes more than that—maybe it takes ten thousand. But if you keep practicing the required skill, eventually you will become competent at it. At this stage skill is present, but consciousness is not yet developed. You know that you can do it, but do not know why it works. Some people take the other route. They are going to learn everything there is to know about adjusting (or about marketing and attracting new patients to their practice). They are going to read every book there is, they are going to take every course there is. They are just going to know what it takes to adjust an L4, L5 facet correctly, and why it will work. They will not yet be able to do it until they have practiced. Clearly there are two paths from amateur to pro.

In reality, none of us takes one way or the other, rather we take a zigzag course. We think we would like to do something so we try it a few times, that is practice. Then we wonder why it works, and we read something or talk to somebody. That's development of consciousness. And then we return to practice the setup and thrust some more and we become more effective and efficient at it. We become better at the particular skill. We are all in the process of developing from amateur to pro status, a continuous, circuitous effort.

Earlier we congratulated you. To stay with the pro football analogy, it appears to us that you are the player, and we have been asked to assist you in developing the game plan and the preparation for execution. We are honored by the request, and trust that the following will help you. Remember, your actions, procedures, protocols, execution, and care for your patients will be a determining factor in the future of the profession. Let's make sure it is a promising future. Let's assure high-quality service. Let's assure the survival and growth of the chiropractic lifestyle.

2

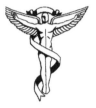 **Management Approaches**

For the well-trained physician, the person who has received an excellent clinical education, the concepts in this text are totally different from those which have been received during professional training. The successful health-care provider is, besides being an excellent physician, also an entrepreneur, a manager, and a business owner. Therefore, knowledge of such areas as marketing, personnel management, accounting, financial planning, negotiating, business law, and insurance are prerequisites to a successful practice.

In this chapter a concept will be presented which can be applied directly to the running of a business by the new physician. In order to supply a frame of reference for the system which follows, or any other system one may wish to use, a small amount of management theory is useful.

Management

Business management texts utilize various ways of categorizing the functions of management. Frequently, the classification takes the form of a listing of functions typically allocated to managers. One might read, for example, the following:

The functions of management are:
- Hiring, firing, and supervising personnel
- Acquisition, utilization, and disposition of capital assets

- Planning and implementation of corporate goals
- Creation of an organizational structure

Another approach used is an all-encompassing statement, such as, "The manager is responsible for running the organization in such a manner that optimal use of capital, people, and property is made."

Starting in the early part of this century, management became a subject of study. Two approaches evolved:

1.   The quantitative (scientific) approach, which considers all management decisions to be quantifiable and, as a consequence, promotes the elimination of risk in running a business.

2.   The behavioral approach, which considers management to be a sociological phenomenon, and therefore applies the laws of sociology in a business environment and in managing an organization. The behavioralists recognize that, besides group factors, individual attitudes and actions also have an effect on organizations and, therefore, the precepts of psychology are useful in the study of management as well.

In today's management circles the above approaches are referred to by the shorthand designations of Theory X and Theory Y. Theory X holds that the human being is by nature not interested in work. The Theory X manager must, therefore, strictly control and supervise the worker. Theory Y holds almost the opposite belief: human beings seek their fulfillment through work and are by nature interested in doing right, learning, and making progress. All the Theory Y manager has to do is provide the correct atmosphere.

It was not until the middle of this century that management students started realizing that both of the above approaches reflect the real world in part. From the apparent diversity of the two approaches came a third theory, one frequently called the integrated management theory, sometimes referred to as Theory Z. Reading texts espousing the integrated management theory, one might find this definition of management: "Management is the planning, organizing, directing, and controlling of businesses so that the objectives of the group, and all individuals in it, can be achieved in the most economical and effective manner."

Business courses rarely address the unique problems of service industries. The management of professional practices is not discussed at all. Only very recently have a small number of articles and books been written to assist the business owner in the health-care professions. Most of the authors are practicing professionals with a few years' experience behind them. This literature addresses the problems of running a medical practice, a law office, or a chiropractic clinic. Typically, little theoretical background is provided. These practical authors appear to feel that, since their experience was acquired empirically, there is no benefit to having supporting theory prior to actually starting the practice. Clearly these authors have little understanding of the concepts presented in Chapter 1: Professionals are conscious, competent persons. They are competent but have not yet arrived at a level of consciousness that allows them to be good mentors and teachers. They probably believe that imitation is enough. The thought, "I was successful this way, so you must be successful in the same manner," does not recognize the reality that not all entrepreneurs fit the profile.

Without a conceptual framework, theories are not very helpful in assisting the starting entrepreneur to increase his potential for success. We will try to provide a conceptual framework which will allow professionals to create their own systems for running a business without feeling as if they are the first ones ever to struggle with the problems normally encountered in starting a business.

PPBIC

The conceptual framework to be employed is entitled PPBIC (Planning, Programming, Budgeting, Implementation, Control). It is not intended as a step-by-step process, but rather as a set of concepts which assist the entrepreneur in understanding the functions of management. PPBIC is not new; in fact, the first three steps had a high public profile in the Department of Defense during the Kennedy Administration. Secretary McNamara, a former president of the Ford Motor Company and still a young man when he was named secretary of defense, brought a new approach to the budgetary system. He introduced Planning, Programming, and Budgeting as a system to the federal government, and thus to the world. We have added Implementation and Control, to create a complete concept of management's functions. A short discussion will aid in the understanding of these five terms.

Planning

Planning can be defined as stating the objectives of the business owner, in broad terms, for the type of practice, market, and geographic location in which the office will exist. The time horizon is long-term, three to five years, and, as a result, the planning statements are of necessity vague or "fuzzy" and flexible. An example for a recently graduated physician could be: "I will own and operate a clinic in one of the new, growing suburbs of a large metropolitan area in the temperate climate zone of the United States. This clinic will have a moderate patient count, specialize in pediatric care, generate an income my family can live on comfortably, allow me to pursue my hobbies as well as my family life, and allow for travel on a quarterly basis." The result of this planning process should be the vision and mission statements and the list of critical needs to be used by the business to provide the requisite long-term focus for success.

Programming

Programming is the activity immediately following planning. It requires a narrower definition of statements made in the planning portion. Programming creates the steps necessary to achieve the plan as stated. Obviously, choices will have to be made during this activity. It is also the first time a prospective entrepreneur comes in contact with risk evaluation. Programming requires the filling in of details not earlier considered and the creation of measuring sticks for recognizing when goals in the plan have been accomplished. Creating specific time frames is a part of the programming activity. Time frames are much shorter than in the planning stage, and, as a result, much more inflexible and better defined. For example, the date of opening needs to be determined, and all necessary work needs to be scheduled. In Chapter 4 a handy tool will be introduced for this phase: the Critical Path visual.

To further develop the plan started above, some choices now have to be made. A choice of geographic locations must be made, for instance, Kansas City, Minneapolis, Milwaukee, San Francisco, and Louisville would all meet the requirements. Decisions about how to start the business need to be made: Will I start from scratch? Will I buy an existing practice? Will I join an existing practice as an associate or partner? Other typical programming decisions include these: What is a comfortable income? How much work time is comfortable? Can family life be integrated with unusual office hours? What are the continuing education requirements? Can seminar and course attendance be integrated with family vacation and travel plans? There will be many others.

Budgeting

Budgeting is the activity of allocating financial resources to the specific steps indicated by programming. In this stage, cash-flow analyses, pro forma income statements, and balance sheets will be created. The budget thus created becomes the financial plan for the chosen time period. Budgeting, as used in this text, is always a financial/monetary activity. The colloquial concept of "budgeting time" will here be thought of as part of programming. In Chapter 4 an explanation of multilevel budgeting will be introduced. It is referred to as ABC budgeting.

Implementation

Implementation is the actual execution of the work planned, programmed, and budgeted for. Many entrepreneurs discover during implementation that everything that needs to be done takes more time and costs more money than originally expected. Therefore, they learn to be conservative in their expectations. This means they purposefully underestimate new-patient counts, fees for services and collections, and overestimate expenses and time necessary to accomplish a task. A good rule of thumb, which is applicable to any startup or change situation, is: If you think it will cost so much, double it, and if you think will take so long, double that too.

Control

Control is a check of the progress being made. Actual results are compared with plans, programs, and budgets. It is a continuous activity. Specific attention is paid to what is transpiring in the business to assure that the effort expended yields the result desired. Like a driver's control of the car during a trip, progress control requires constant vigilance about the minute changes occurring every moment. Business owners often set aside particular times to have review sessions. These can be scheduled regularly at "dead times" at the office, or as special occasions for staff meetings away from the office. It is difficult to generalize about frequency of such review sessions, as much depends on the needs of the owner and the employees. The stage of development of the business also affects the timing of regular and special discussions.

In order to effectively control the growth and development of the practice, record-keeping and development of operational statistics is required. Without measuring sticks, it is impossible to gauge progress. In appendices A, B, and C we provide some samples of helpful statistics and their graphic representation.

Many entrepreneurs will identify a success to congratulate the staff on, as a positive lead-in for review discussions. Nothing is wrong with celebrating the accomplishment of even the smallest objective. Everyone likes to receive a pat on the back in recognition of an achievement. This approach has the advantage of putting the entrepreneur and staff in a positive frame of mind, resulting in a better attitude. Controls of processes and insistence on adherence to standards and protocol are a prerequisite for the success of a business. These do not have to be negative and should, in fact, be quite productive and positive.

Once the planning, programming, and budgeting steps are completed and implementation has started, "the plan" should be considered as cast in concrete. Changes should be made only after the control function shows unequivocally that the "mistake" is indeed in the plan and not in the implementation. Too often, when things do not develop as planned, a quick decision is made that the plan was wrong and should be changed. Most of the time, the plan is fine but the implementation was not executed as originally envisioned. Only when it is clear that the implementation is correct, should consideration of a change in plan, program, and budget follow.

Finally, the individual who can be effective in reviewing results alone is rather rare. Most entrepreneurs find the old cliché, "Two heads are better than one," is excellent advice when it is critical review time.

From these short descriptions of the PPBIC steps, it is obvious that this process is not a one-time activity. Instead, a conceptual framework for the management of a business has been provided to the entrepreneur. It can be used effectively during various stages in the life of the business.

Moral of the story: PPBIC is a continuous and circuitous activity for the entrepreneur. It does not allow for the creation of a plan which, upon completion, will reside in the bottom left-hand drawer of the desk, never to see the light of day again. *Planning, Programming, Budgeting, Implementation,* and *Control* are the basic steps of management.

Management By Objective

Earlier in this chapter, three theoretical management approaches were presented—scientific, behavioral, and integrationist—the latter approach including the concept of Management By Objective (MBO) as a tool to implement the theory. PPBIC translates MBO to the small professional practice. It is helpful to understand how MBO works in a large business before attempting to apply it in PPBIC terms to a professional practice. A humorous but realistic review will help.

Let us assume that we are looking into the windows of XYZ Corporation, the famous widget manufacturer mentioned in all economics texts. We notice in the office of the president a meeting of the senior officers of the corporation. The chairman of the board of directors (BOD) is leading the discussion in his capacity as chief executive officer (CEO), depending upon the president, who is the chief operating officer (COO), for appropriate assistance. It appears the BOD executive committee has laid out a strategic five-year plan for XYZ which will require the doubling of sales and profits. (The senior vice president for finance interrupts, saying, for the uninitiated, that this means an annual compound growth rate of 15 percent. We should realize that growth at XYZ in the past has been around 5 percent per year.) In other words, the BOD is requiring a highly ambitious change in corporate movement. The CEO finishes his part of the discussion by stating that he is certain that this fine senior management team will find the way to accomplish these objective. He impresses upon each of them the importance of each department's creating its own program for implementation (to accomplish its part in support of the overall organization). He then strongly encourages some brainstorming to arrive at a program. Some discussion follows, and usually a decision is made not to follow the more traditional route the manager would have taken, but to try this new and open planning approach. This runs quite contrary to the route the traditional manger would prefer to take: close the office door, put pen to paper, and write memos to the immediate subordinates dictating their actions. The organization will undergo a lot of stress as a result of trying this new approach, but stress has a creative component.

Clearly, we are looking through the windows of an integrationist's office. We need to be aware that each of the senior management people who has just listened to the chairman of the BOD's speech arrived at the current position only through twenty or more years of hard work, first as a technician of some kind, later as a technical supervisor (probably most of the twenty-plus years were spent here), and only very recently as head of a department. This is important, because this sort of manager is accustomed to telling people what to do, rather than asking them what they would like to do. It is also the habit of these managers to follow the boss's lead. The result of following this person's lead is known as "the trickle-down effect," or to put it another way, "an organization becomes a reflection of the person at the top."

As good leaders who learned by following, the senior management team members disperse to their own offices to implement the instructions provided. Now, the trickle-down effect and Murphy's Law (whatever can go wrong, will) work in cooperation with each other, assuring that by the time MBO arrives on the desk of the recently hired nineteen-year-old typist, or the janitor, or any person at the low end of the totem pole, everybody is totally confused as to the intent of the instructions. Many meetings between individual employees and their supervisors are scheduled. During these, each employee accepts responsibility for performing certain tasks, in a certain manner, within a given time frame. Discussions are often confused, sometimes heated, because MBO requires honest, open communication between supervisor and subordinate. While such communication exists commonly in other countries, businesses in the United States have not been managed with quite such democratic openness.

A few months later, looking again through the windows of the XYZ president's office, we arrive at the conclusion that, to everybody's surprise, a reasonable amount of work has been accomplished by all. Appropriate budgetary figures are established, which, should implementation be accomplished as planned and control appropriately exercised, come within a hairsbreadth of accomplishing the goals the executive committee of the BOD pulled out of thin air some time ago. Now converted to the integrationist style, the management team throws a party for itself to celebrate the acceptance of modern management behavior in the company.

Conclusion

While purposefully oversimplified, this story describes the introduction of MBO into many American businesses. It demonstrates that Management By Objective is derived from a combination of the scientific and behaviorist schools of management thought, which have been integrated into one useful system. The question now becomes: How does the sole practitioner, or the managing partner responsible for the running of a small organization, utilize this cumbersome time-consuming, paper-intensive approach to the running of the business? The answer lies in utilizing the concepts, rather than every detail of the system. We have attempted to provide these concepts in our explanation of PPBIC.

Since the early 1960s, when Emerson Electric first introduced MBO to the world of business, much has been learned by managers and academics. Today we have the knowledge of organizational and human behavior to realize that the basic ingredients require some assistance from the concepts of team dynamics and organizational change agents. Appendix I, the list of resources, provides some excellent sources for additional information and learning.

3

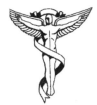

Startup and Marketing

Before we provide a list of some specific things to do in the day-to-day running of the practice, some background thoughts on marketing of the practice are in order. As indicated in Chapter 1, we know of no chiropractor who thought, Hey, I love to sell and do marketing work, why don't I go to chiropractic school? In fact the opposite is frequently the case: people who have a desire to serve others, who may become excited about some aspect of human life that they feel they can improve for themselves and others, or people who have a desire for deep scientific understanding of the human body—these are the people who enter the health-care fields. Chiropractic is no different, it attracts the same kind of individuals.

And yet, as Tom Peters and others have so clearly indicated over the last few years, any business without the proper customer-oriented attitude will not long survive in the later part of the twentieth century. If we analyze the factors determining success for a chiropractic practice, we quickly realize that the cornerstone is the ability of the practice to attract patients. Without new patients, there is no one to provide health care to. Therefore, no fees can be charged for services, no collections can be made on those fees, no moneys are available to pay the office expenses, or the employee salaries, or the doctor's (read: owner's) profit to take home. It all starts with getting the prospective patient to come into the office for care.

We can already hear the reaction: "Well, providing good care is all I need to do to bring patients in." Our reaction is simple: No, it is *not*. First, if we assume the reader intends to start a practice from scratch, where does the first patient come from? Second, if an existing practice does not have a continuous influx of new patients, how are the patients who die or move out of the area going to be replaced? And third, what about patients who do not have the chiropractic attitude, who are still so immersed in our allopathic or Newtonian society, who indicate all they want is symptomatic relief and then disappear from your practice forever?

All professionals, at least those with professional ethics, provide high-quality service and have the best interest of their client or patient at heart. It will be these who can expect to eventually obtain a good-sized portion of their new patients through referrals from existing patients. Many of those existing patients, though, will require a little nudge, a little reminder, such as, "We are glad to accept new patients in the practice; do you know anyone who would benefit from seeing us?" Therefore, no matter what stage of the life cycle the practice is in, marketing and new patient acquisition are prerequisites for success of the practice.

The textbooks employed in marketing courses will define the term in the first or second chapter: Marketing is the discipline dealing with the four *P's:*

1. Product
2. Place and distribution
3. Price
4. Promotion

In our estimation, for a professional office, the promotion factor is the one which really counts. Product is rather clearly defined, although young practitioners need to spend time and attention on defining and delineating it. Place, we feel, is rather immaterial because of the nature of the doctor-patient relationship. Price seems to be no great concern; even with managed care organizations firmly established in the health-care field, chiropractors are rarely questioned on the level of fees. Promotion, then, is the factor we need to pay attention to.

Promotion should be viewed from two distinct perspectives: patient retention and patient acquisition. The first perspective is comprised of those efforts directed at maintaining the present patient population as clients and assisting them in referring new patients. The second perspective deals with bringing in new people, who have no connection to the practice, as patients. A fact of life for the chiropractor is the effort of building a practice based on the doctor-patient relationship. This relationship, in turn, is built on trust. Trust can only be developed through personal exposure of one person to the other over a period of time. Advertising—a component of marketing, not a synonym for marketing—cannot do for a chiropractor's office what it can do for the sale of cereal from the grocery store. We have all heard the wisdom of marketing consultants, of the yellow pages advertising salesperson, of the coupon and group direct-mail experts, but we should maintain a good level of skepticism toward any message that says, "I can bring you patients without your personal involvement," when the basis of the relationship is personal trust.

Because of the typical attitude and background of the chiropractor, some basic concepts of sales and marketing are appropriate. Our friends Mr. Bill Esteb and Dr. Rob Jackson, owners of BackTalk Systems, Inc., do a very fine job teaching chiropractors about patient education (their term), much better then we could do here. Others also address this topic quite well. A few thoughts on acquiring patients, though, seem in order.

The Selling Process

Just as there are myths about entrepreneurs, so are there myths about selling. Some of the most pervasive myths seem to be that selling is not professional and that salesmen are born, not made. Quite the contrary is true. We have all witnessed some salespeople in action and judged them to be excellent professionals. Besides, lawyers, architects, engineers, and accountants all have to sell to obtain clients, just as doctors have to sell to obtain patients. When observing professional salespersons, one arrives quickly at the realization that this professional is not "born to the manner" (pun intended). These professionals have learned and studied and practiced to arrive at the level of the professional. Attending seminars on selling for some of these professionals leads to some basic concepts we can all use and internalize through practice. They strongly believe in and apply the counselor selling approach and its sales cycle. Dr. Ronald Kelemen, the chief of staff of Logan College Health Centers, helped us put it into chiropractese:

New Patient Contact Cycle (we still call it the sales cycle)

1. Meet the public (John and Jane Q.).
2. Qualify them for potential patient status (answer the following three questions):
   a. Can I show this individual a need for chiropractic?
   b. Is the individual approachable, physically and mentally?

   c. Can the individual afford the cost of the care I will propose?

3. A prospective patient exists only if all three questions are positively answered.

4. Develop, in your professional opinion, a specific need for chiropractic care.

5. Obtain the prospect's agreement to the need (remember "need" is your professional judgment, "want" is the prospective patient's way of expressing thoughts that may be less correct). In other words, marry the want to the need.

6. Only after obtaining the prospect's agreement, offer the solution: your services.

7. Once the patient's condition is improving, take the time to ask for referrals.

The authors are convinced that if the above process is followed in a step-by-step fashion, even individuals who start out being skeptical about you and chiropractic can successfully be brought into the world of quality health care. Rushing through the process only leads to disappointment. If you find an individual whom you have brought to Step 6, objecting to your solution to their wants and needs, you should return to Step 5 and maybe to Step 3.

Practice-building is an ongoing process. It needs to be conscious as well as subconscious; both the doctor and staff are needed to establish and maintain patient relationships. The correct, customer-oriented attitude needs to show in thought and action in all areas of the practice. Factors such as professional and thorough care, awareness of the patient as an individual with feelings, smooth office functions, and up-to-date knowledge by the physician and staff, are indispensable. This attitude will cause patients to be confident enough in the practice to refer others.

The Owner's Role

The owner's role in a practice is, in addition to providing health care, to be the leader. It is necessary for the entrepreneur to set goals, be motivated, develop standards, and stay focused. If one is enthusiastic and productive, these attitudes will be conveyed to the staff, patients, and community.

When not with patients, which will occur rather frequently in the beginning, there is much that can be done—learn more about your patients, work on practice-building ideas, read professional journals. Not only is this productive time for the practice, but it also sets an excellent example for the staff. You cannot ask more of them than you ask of yourself.

Effective Leadership

The owner is the only one, initially, who can provide the required leadership. The vision of the owner must be shared, first with the staff, then with the patients. Only in this manner can the vision permeate the organization, and from there, the entire community. Take time to understand the people around you. This needs to include both patients and staff. Effective leadership is built on mutual respect. Make the patients and staff feel important. The desire to feel important is a strong human trait. Things you can do to make people feel important and raise their level of self-esteem are:

- Be a skillful listener. Let them talk. Watch body language. Pause and think before answering.
- Compliment.
- Use their names. Concentrate on the "you," not the "me."
- Acknowledge them. If patients have been waiting (which should happen only rarely), let them know that you are aware of their time obligations. When staff are reliable, do good work, are dependable, do tasks beyond the "call of duty," acknowledge them.
- Be gracious.
- Agree when possible, admit when wrong.

Things you can do to show that you value your staff:

- Ask their opinions.
- Fulfill your office responsibilities. If a staff person needs a report completed, do it. Don't wait to be pestered for it.
- Support openly the responsibility of your staff.
- Have weekly staff meetings. Making a contribution is part of creating the feeling of being involved and responsible to your role.

To be an effective leader, concentrate on the positive and promote it publicly. Be realistic in your expectations and reward performance that meets the standard—yours, your staff's, and that of your patients. Avoid having a negative attitude. It takes a very conscious effort to be positive, but it is infectious to others.

Developing Yourself

A necessity for developing a successful practice, and sustaining it once achieved, is to have proper estimation of your self worth. An internal belief and strength must be developed. By understanding yourself and what your needs are, you can transfer that inner strength outward toward your practice. If you have a progressive, focused momentum, your practice will align itself with that momentum. Develop yourself internally first. Use the following guidelines to help you in forming your internal strengths and values:

- Make your mental attitude positive, supportive, goal-directed, open. Control your thoughts to avoid fear and panic. Remain focused on your vision and mission.
- Set goals and keep reaching higher as each one is attained.
- Take a salary (doctor's draw). Keep your practice as financially stable as possible. If you fluctuate from high-income weeks to low-income weeks, and you pay yourself the balance, you'll keep the practice on unstable ground.
- Read professional journals, and attend seminars. You must keep abreast of all new developments and trends in the profession and in health care, generally.
- Be active in all aspects of your life and practice. If you sit and wait for action to come your way, your practice will reflect this attitude.
- Learn humility without humbling yourself.
- Don't take on an apologetic manner toward patients for their care. If in your judgment they need x-rays or therapy, emphasize the rationale. You are there to give them the best service possible.
- You represent what you want your practice to be. You must lead by example.
- Focus is the key word, it is what makes successful people successful.

Once you have developed internal strength, there are steps you can take to help others view you as a professional:

- Remember you are a doctor, a professional. Dress and conduct yourself in a professional manner. Wear a suit and tie or business dress to meetings. In your office, wear a tie and clinic jacket or business dress and clinic coat. Remember the effect the image you present has on others.

- Carry your business cards and hand them out.
- Introduce yourself to the local professional community.
- Join community organizations and be an active member. Being a name on a list helps neither you nor the organization.
- Don't compromise your practice philosophy or mechanics of practice to overcome a preceding doctor's reputation.
- Be on time! Everyone's time is valuable.
- Make eye contact. It implies you are comfortable with and acknowledge the other person.
- Be as active and enthusiastic in your professional life as you are in your personal life. Your personal life will depend on it.
- Promote your local social and business community.
- Be involved.

Promoting Your Practice

Practice-building requires an ongoing conscious effort. It does not stop once you have established your practice. More than half of any growth in the practice will come from patient-retention strategies. The majority of this comes from patient referrals. The rest of your practice increase will come from the promotion of your practice. Start with community involvement. Buy goods and services locally when possible. Join local civic organizations such as the Jaycees, Optimists, Lions, the chamber of commerce, a church, a youth group, a hobby group. If you are involved, you will become known and recognized for your contributions to society. Volunteer to give community health and wellness talks. Be active in school activities; for example, be a sports team doctor. Community involvement is the most positive way to have your name become known, to create what advertisers call: "top-of-the-mind awareness" of you and your business.

There are several ways to keep your practice visible without appearing to be soliciting. All can be done with the utmost taste and at the same time will educate the public about the benefits of chiropractic. For example:

- Signage: Design a well-recognized sign to identify your office site.
- Newspaper articles: Develop a series of brief articles explaining common health problems and what chiropractic can accomplish with them.
- Direct mailings: Send out newsletters and educational articles to the community and patients.

- Mall shows: Health fairs are often promoted in local communities, especially malls.
- Yellow pages: Put a lot of thought into your ad layout. This will offer the public insight into your practice. Be very professional and informative. Do not clutter up your ad copy.
- Newspaper ads: Until your practice appears in the phone book, you might consider having an ad in the newspaper. Keep it professional and simple.

Networking

Networking allows every new business owner to develop contacts that will further his or her professional development. The people on this list and/or the business or organizations that they represent will serve as a referral base, and you will refer others to them. Thus the network becomes a mutual support and admiration society, a true win-win-win for you, the other networker, and the mutual client or patient.

Patient Relations

No matter how many years you have been in practice, you must promote good public relations with your current and prospective patients. Send out "new patient" letters, "thank you for referring" letters, holiday cards, or newsletters. Provide literature updates for patients to read. Educational pamphlets can be given to patients each time at check-in or check-out. Commercial firms, such as BackTalk Systems and others, have prepared some excellent pieces for your use. Those may be acquired at very reasonable costs.

If your work is not improving the patient's condition, don't hesitate to get a second opinion. Or if the patient needs another specialty, refer out. Not only is it the correct way to treat the patient, it will also validate you as a caring doctor in the eyes of other health care providers, specialists, and the patient.

Because, eventually, a high percentage of new patients will come from patient referrals, it makes sense to treat your patients well. There are many things you can do to show your patients you value them:

- Think service above all else. If you put the dollar first, it will show in your attitude and actions.
- Call acute patients to determine how they are progressing. This can be done by you or your staff. Designate who is to be respon-

sible and identify who should be called. It is a great service and provides excellent public relations. People will be surprised and pleased that you actually called.

	Name	Address	Phone
Bank			
Accountant			
Attorney			
Medical Doctors			
Family			
Orthopedist			
Neurologist			
Radiologist			
Dentist			
Laboratory			
Local Chiropractors			
Hospital			
Administrator			
City Government			
School			
Civic Groups			
Newspaper			
Radio			

Fig. 3.1. A master form will assist you in building a personal and professional network.

- Use high-quality time with each patient. Each patient is an individual. Some patients will require more time than others.
- Create a present-time consciousness with each patient visit. When you are with patients, focus totally on them. Do not think about how far behind you are. Stay focused in your conversations; do not divert to your last golf game.
- Develop trust; begin by keeping your word. Develop sincerity, follow-through, keep your promises to your patients.
- Be there for your patients, even if you run a few minutes late or start a few minutes early. Set hours that will serve the patients—maybe an evening a week, or Saturday mornings. You may see only two or three patients, but the patients know you are there.
- Treat all patients with the same high standard of respect, regardless of their appearance or social level.

Difficult Patients

You will find that patients often have a clear idea of their treatment needs in spite of your professional advice. You must recognize that this is normal and know how to deal with it. As indicated earlier, when the new patient contact cycle was introduced, it may be necessary for you to reestablish the need and want combination which originally convinced the patient to come to you for care. All patients have the potential to provide referrals, but you must earn the right to receive those. One negative comment will spread faster than ten positive ones.

There will be patients in your practice whom you cannot please; as soon as you recognize the patient as this kind of individual, refer him or her to a provider who is better suited to the patient's style and personality. Recognize that there is no fault to be found in this situation, the patient deserves the best possible health care, but due to a personality conflict between the two of you, you cannot provide it. You cannot convince people they need care if they believe otherwise. You will not be able to please everyone, and trying to do so will cause you more frustration than it is worth. Work with the patients who want your help. Follow through with the agreed upon care programs. Patients who receive more than they expect are the ones who will refer. You must get a commitment from patients to cooperate and follow through with their care plans. If they are positive about themselves, they will be positive about the care you have given them.

Patient Retrieval Procedures

Acquiring new patients is expensive in terms of time, energy, and money; satisfied former patients make excellent "new" patients. It is wise, therefore, to develop a patient retrieval procedure. Patients drop from care for various reasons. Forget those whom you know to be "lost." Contact patients whom you have not seen in a long time, or designate an assistant to follow through periodically for you. Occasional "social" calls may lead to the discovery of new conditions or recurring old ones.

The following sample portion of a telephone conversation illustrates a good way to reactivate a patient.

Office: Mrs. Johnson, have you thought of discussing this problem with the doctor?

Patient: Actually, I was thinking of calling the office for an appointment.

Office: Would Monday or Tuesday be best?

Patient: Tuesday would work better for me.

Office: (Give choice of time) Which is better for you?

Other Things You Can Do to Build Your Practice

Another practice development technique is maintaining a statistics sheet. Keep records of your performance and develop statistics to help you to set goals. As most people have an easier time interpreting pictures rather then tables, create graphs. Post this where only you and your staff have access—patients might get the wrong impression about your attitude if it is displayed in a patient access area. Let the staff be involved with the tracking of statistics. This provides an incentive for involvement. Set the statistics sheet up on daily and monthly bases, transferring that information to the yearly form. It is amazing how seeing the numbers in black and white allows you to see growth that you may not have felt was there.

Make sure your personnel are positive, cheerful, dedicated to your practice and philosophy, and that they are willing to do what is needed to make the practice grow. Encourage your staff to schedule a full day of appointments; the prospect of leaving work early shouldn't override patient service. When a patient calls for an appointment, get that patient in. It will become very evident if a staff person is there only for the paycheck. Don't tolerate this type of behavior; correct it.

In addition, you can build your practice if you:
- Provide a brochure on the practice and doctor;
- Send out a questionnaire inquiring about the services of the practice;
- Offer a "welcome certificate," offering the new patient a complimentary consultation and exam;
- Associate with successful people.

Part Two

Basic Business Concerns

4

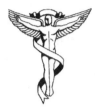 **Planning
Requirements**

A number of clichés exist to remind us of the important part planning plays in our lives. The authors are partial to this one: "People do not plan to fail, they simply fail to plan." It makes clear the fact that a plan is crucial if one wishes to exert some control over one's destination in life. In the planning process, if executed correctly, foresight and insight are developed.

Academicians, students of human behavior and organization, have long identified a series of steps in developing a plan. Well-designed business plans contain six levels of thought:

1. Vision
2. Mission
3. Goals
4. Objectives
5. Strategies
6. Action steps

A vision is a clarion call to the one seeing it. It is a fuzzy, way-out-there kind of understanding. It is sometimes hard to put into words, even harder to write down. Frequently, individuals who have a vision of what they want their practice to be like, when asked to present it to another, will stumble, talk fragmentedly about some things and concepts, and then in frustration will finish with a paraphrase of the old definition of art: "I can't describe it, but I'll know it when I have achieved it." A mission statement is a more definitive statement of the reason for being of the organization. It is rather specific and is most often stated using action words and phrases. Together the vision and the mission statements provide the long-term guidance required during the busy, confusing start-up period of the practice. They become the touchstone for the planning and implementation processes later, when day-to-day activities have a way of requiring total attention and the long-term vision is obscured in the fog of activity. Having frequent reminders to one's self of the vision and the mission are crucial at those times; they help one avoid drifting and help handle the challenges presented in running a practice. If the vision is achieved, the mission has been accomplished. Ethics, the personal and professional values underlying our actions, should be a part of the vision as well as the mission.

Goals are broad statements of the accomplishments intended to be achieved. They are still rather broad and far into the future. Objectives are the shorter-term goal statements that are more precise and can become the measuring sticks, the milestones along the way, used to assure that the route taken leads to the objective intended. The goal, in turn, must support the traveler and lead to the accomplishment of the vision. Strategies are the specific routes designed to accomplish first the goal, next the objectives, and finally the vision. Action steps are the very specific steps designed, in combination or sequentially, to implement the strategy, which will lead to the objective to accomplish the goal.

Many of our acquaintances do not like to take the time to write this series of, sometimes initially rather fuzzy and disjointed, pages necessary to clarify thinking. In developing a business plan, it is crucial that the entrepreneur take the time to assure the vision, mission, and so on are indeed what is intended. Only time and effort will allow this to happen. We called the process crucial because to be successful in running an entrepreneurial business it is necessary that the entrepreneur try to have a personal design and purpose. Copying someone else's plan is most likely to lead to failure. No one else knows the feelings, the ego income factors, the frustrations, and the desires that the entrepreneur has invested in the plan, and therefore in the vision.

Planning tools abound. Brainstorming and benchmarking are well-known tools. The use of information gathering, decision trees, and such are less commonly referred to; however, all are tools used in planning. A crucial factor, to be recognized in developing a well-designed plan, is that one mind can not conceive of all possible future occurrences. While we do not intend to state that "all bases must be covered at all times," we do wish to remind the reader of the risks and frustrations discussed in Chapter 1. To know that reality will send obstacles our way is to understand the need for alternative approaches to obtaining the objectives. Some of the limitations we humans face in the planning processes are built into us. On the following pages we will deal with three such factors.

Mindset

In this world there is no human being who does not have a mind. It is a wonderful instrument and can be exercised as well as, or better than, the human body. The mind does have limitations, however. A limitation one needs to be aware of is the mindset. The trait of not paying attention to things other than the task at hand may be very positive. In difficult times, when we plow through no matter what the obstacles, we say we have determination. When starting a new business, one requires a large portion of determination.

Mindset can be counterproductive, however, when it stops us from looking at other possibilities when needed. When we are trying to write the business plan, a closed mindset is a hindrance. It stops us from perceiving all possible solutions to the situation being reviewed. It is normal to view a problem from one angle; habit has taught us to remain in a given mindset, and experience has taught us that a certain way of looking at a problem yields usable solutions. In planning a new enterprise, however, the entrepreneur unnecessarily limits the possible viable solutions by remaining within a given mindset. During the planning phase, it is extremely important that a number of different mindsets are used in establishing and reviewing the objectives.

Let us take a moment to look at an example of a mind-set. Without reading below please look at this picture, and write down a few of the thoughts that enter your mind as a result.

Fig. 4.1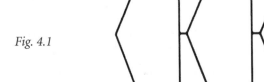

Assuming you have played the game fairly, you certainly have a list of things you see in the above picture. The usual items that will be mentioned when this drawing is presented to a group of people include arrows pointing left, three home plates, houses on their side, bullets, and computer programmer's decision points. Rarely, if ever, does someone in a group suggest what was intended to be seen here: two capital letter *K*'s.

Once this is suggested, though, one can hear recognition move through the entire group. The individual mentioning the *K* has changed the mindset for everyone in the group by suggesting, "Look between the pictures." A followup exercise immediately yields a chorus of shouts:

Fig. 4.2

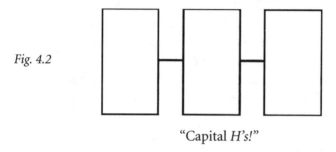

"Capital *H's!*"

The moral of this exercise is that to change your mindset, assistance from other people is probably needed. It is extremely important for the entrepreneur to be aware of tunnel vision and mindset while in the writing phase of the business plan. It is possible, but difficult, to change your own mindset. You can deal with this phenomenon by changing topics under consideration frequently, or by leaving the work and returning later with a fresh mindset. Probably the best approach is to have another person review your work and bring a new mindset.

The Critical Path

People who plan things discover one of two things: either there is never enough time to do what needs to be done, or all stages follow logically and smoothly one after the other. In the construction industry a tool exists which can assure that a project runs as scheduled: the Critical Path. Minor adaptation can make this "Critical Path" approach useful for any planning endeavor.

All tasks to be accomplished prior to opening the office have a certain time frame in which they can be accomplished. In addition, some tasks cannot be begun until other tasks are completed. In other words, tasks must be accomplished in a certain order. As an example, a senior in chiropractic college, starting to plan for opening an office in Jefferson City, Missouri, must graduate, pass the national and state boards, find the right office location, have leasehold improvements completed, and the like. How can all this run smoothly?

In the diagram on the next page (figure 4.3), durations are assigned to each of the tasks. Some tasks can be worked on simultaneously, others can only be accomplished sequentially. The time anticipated for completion is indicated by the length of the line between the points. All lines running horizontally indicate tasks which may be worked on simultaneously. Tasks to the right cannot be started until the ones to the left are finished. This approach is frequently enhanced with color coding. Red is usually saved for the path that cannot be delayed if the office is to be opened on time. This is the Critical Path, and deserves attention at all times. Because it is a visual aid, many starting entrepreneurs find the Critical Path diagram to be extremely helpful.

ABC Budgeting

Part of planning is the creation of alternatives. Organizations frequently refer to a second alternative as Plan B. Large multinational corporations sometimes have a problem predicting how well a new product will be received by consumers. These corporations solve that dilemma by using ABC budgeting.

Professionals starting a practice need to be careful with cash flow in the early stages of operation. An adaptation of ABC budgeting can help to create alternate plans at the same time. Let's assume we are trying to decide how often to place a certain advertisement in the local weekly newspaper and how many assistants are needed for the smooth running of the office. ABC budgeting concepts would suggest three different expenditure levels. The determination of which level will actually be implemented is made by the new-patient count over the first three months of operating the clinic. The expenditures are labeled low, medium, and high, or A, B, and C. For the first three months Plan B, or medium, is used; then, based on the new-patient count, advertising and staffing is changed to the A (low) or C (high) plan as indicated. Of course if the new-patient count happens to hit right at that predicted for the medium level, no change in advertising and personnel budget is made. This process is continued quarterly, and quick switches are possible because the work was done during the planning phase of PPBIC.

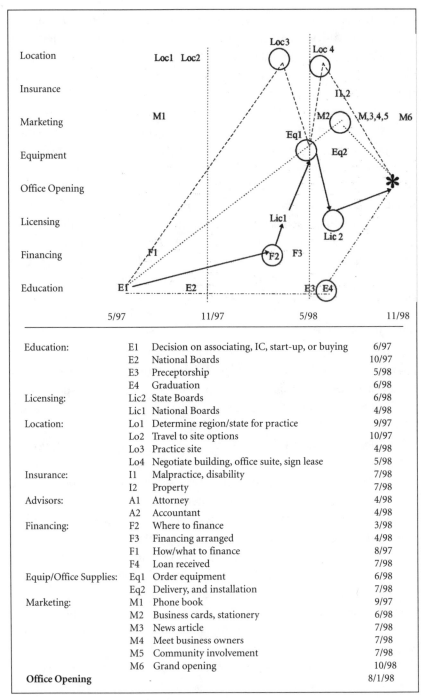

	E1	Decision on associating, IC, start-up, or buying	6/97
Education:	E1	Decision on associating, IC, start-up, or buying	6/97
	E2	National Boards	10/97
	E3	Preceptorship	5/98
	E4	Graduation	6/98
Licensing:	Lic2	State Boards	6/98
	Lic1	National Boards	4/98
Location:	Lo1	Determine region/state for practice	9/97
	Lo2	Travel to site options	10/97
	Lo3	Practice site	4/98
	Lo4	Negotiate building, office suite, sign lease	5/98
Insurance:	I1	Malpractice, disability	7/98
	I2	Property	7/98
Advisors:	A1	Attorney	4/98
	A2	Accountant	4/98
Financing:	F2	Where to finance	3/98
	F3	Financing arranged	4/98
	F1	How/what to finance	8/97
	F4	Loan received	7/98
Equip/Office Supplies:	Eq1	Order equipment	6/98
	Eq2	Delivery, and installation	7/98
Marketing:	M1	Phone book	9/97
	M2	Business cards, stationery	6/98
	M3	News article	7/98
	M4	Meet business owners	7/98
	M5	Community involvement	7/98
	M6	Grand opening	10/98
Office Opening			8/1/98

Fig. 4.3. Critical path illustration.

While the above example describes the use of ABC budgeting for only two expenses, advertising and staffing, in real life all expenses are budgeted in this manner. The income (fees for services and/or collections, in the case of a physician's office) is also projected at the three levels. In this manner, the control function needs to determine only the actual income level, and the expenditure decisions are then automatic. This approach saves heartburn for the entrepreneur at some future time, and it impresses the accountant and—more important—the banker with the physician's thorough understanding of management.

Backwards Thinking

Many individuals have trouble selecting one of the many routes available to a certain destination. In addition, when considering the factors involved in starting a business, questions of optimal route, both from a financial and time perspective, tend to predominate. The authors have found a particular approach useful in these situations: backwards thinking—as in backwards from the future. The process is simple but does require some getting used to. Most of us, when planning, think *forward*. We start by making sure we know where we are, project where we want to be, and then, from the present, design the route to the objective. The backwards thinking approach starts at the objective and looks back to the current situation. We find that using this approach makes it less difficult to "see" the route that allowed us to arrive at the destination. We can, in fact, see a number of ways we could have achieved the "goal" location. Looking back allows us to see the efficiencies of finance and time factor issues. In working with a goodly number of graduates, this approach has proven to be helpful in clearly delineating the vision statement. It is as if the new practitioner can "feel" what it is like to have a thriving practice five years from now. The advantage, then, is that when the actual implementation comes close to the objective, a sense of déjà vu exists to provide comfort and guidance. This approach will allow the entrepreneur to "finish off" the tasks and achieve the ultimate goal. We wish we could take credit for the approach, but it truly belongs to sports psychologists who, working originally with Olympic champions, developed the technique of "visualization."

5

Business Structures

There are three different business structures in use in the United States. The words are commonly used—*proprietorship, partnership,* and *corporation*—but their meaning is not always clear. In everyday language it is not unusual to hear someone say, "I will discuss that with my partner," when in reality there is no partner but rather another stockholder in a closely held corporation. One also hears a sole stockholder describe her- or himself as self-employed, giving the impression that he or she owns a proprietorship

It is not our intent to change the colloquial use of English, but the owner of a business should be able to distinguish between the three forms or structures. He or she should be able to make correct statements about the business's legal form when necessary. Cocktail-partyspeak is not precise enough for all situations.

The significance of the differences between the forms of business structure is in the areas of taxation; liability for the business debts; liability for the actions of the employees; potential for growth for employees; capability (some more apparent than real) to raise capital; control over the operations by the person "in charge"; continuity of the business upon the death of a/ the principal; ease with which the business ownership can be transferred to someone else; legally required actions of surviving partners or personal representatives; and the rights of surviving heirs. A detailed look at each of the business structures will show the effects of these factors.

Proprietorship

The proprietorship is the form of business which is easiest to start and stop and which has the fewest legal requirements.

Starting a proprietorship is as easy as announcing to the world, "I'm open for business." Often this is accomplished simply by ordering business stationery, business cards, and a telephone listing. Until approximately two centuries ago the proprietorship was the manner in which all business was done. Only in recent history has it become the norm to incorporate one's business activities.

Typically, the proprietor's name is included somehow in the name of the business as, for example, "Jones Chiropractic Clinic." Sometimes a fictitious name is used, such as "South Side Clinic." When the owner's name is not used, a filing with the secretary of state of your state is required. In most states this is a minor chore consisting of filling out one form and paying a small filing fee. The purpose of the fictitious-name filing is to provide the general public with easy access to the owner's name and address. Therefore, sometimes on official documents, the term d.b.a. (doing business as) is used. For example, Jeffrey Y. Jones, d.b.a. South Side Clinic.

Legally, the proprietorship has no existence without the owner; it dies when the owner dies. Typically in such cases, a mess is left for the executor (personal representative) to clean up as "liquidating" trustee. Employees who understand this are frequently concerned about their future, especially if the owner is still active at an older age. A potential solution is to make arrangements for transfer of ownership prior to death and to inform the employees. This solution is not foolproof, as disagreement can still easily arise about the assets (honestly, you will learn the meaning of this word) to be included in such a transfer.

From the point of view of federal and state income taxes, the proprietorship is almost as if there is no business. Taxation is accomplished on the owner's individual tax return using one page (called Schedule C for the federal return) to report the financial results of operating the business for the calendar year.

The proprietor is well advised, however, to keep a separate set of books. No one wants the IRS or, worse, the Department of Revenue Sales Tax Bureau, to review all household expenditures when visiting for an audit. Keeping separate books is easy. A checking account at the local bank in the business name is easily established and gives the competent bookkeeper or accountant all the basic information needed for correct recording.

We can chart the advantages and disadvantages of this form of business:

Advantages
- Easy to start
- Low startup costs
- All profits to the owner
- Owner is in total control
- Potentially lower taxation
- Few legal restrictions and regulations
- Easy to stop

Disadvantages
- Unlimited liability (financial and legal)
- Lack of continuity
- Difficult to raise capital
- Limited potential for employees

Partnership

A partnership is also rather simple to start, but more legal requirements exist and display themselves, especially upon dissolution.

There are several types of partnerships:
- *General:* Two or more individuals in business together; each is individually and severally liable for the actions of the partnership, each partner, and each employee.
- *Limited:* By published agreement, the liability of one or more partners is limited. The law requires at least one general (fully liable) partner. This form of partnership is frequently used in investment situations. Typically the limited partner(s) are not involved in the management of the business.
- *Silent:* One or more of the partners is not publicly named. The silent partner may, in fact, be the main one of the organization. More commonly, the silent partner is not at all involved in the business. A silent partner may or may not have limited liability.
- *Nominal:* One or more of the named partners has no ownership interest in the business. Although rarely used, the nominal partnership enhances the prestige of the business by using the nominal partner's name.

Partnerships are started by agreement between the partners to commence business together. This agreement, though not legally required, should be in writing and in enough detail to deal with the common questions which tend to arise in business. Division of initial capital contribution, income, ownership, and management authority are the usual items found in a written partnership agreement. Important to the success of a partnership is the recognition that all decisions will be made by agreement. A partnership agreement may give one partner (the general partner in a limited partnership) the right to make all management decisions.

From the point of view of income tax, the partnership is only a conduit, meaning that while it files federal and state income tax returns, the partnership itself does not pay any federal or state income taxes. This responsibility falls upon the individual partners, who must report their share of business profit on their own tax returns. The tax rate each partner pays is the same as if he or she owned a proprietorship. Any partnership equity (see Chapter 13 for accounting definitions) cannot be withdrawn solely at the whim of the particular partner. To withdraw a portion or all of the partner's capital account requires agreement from the other partners unless specifically allowed in the partnership agreement. Withdrawal of capital severely affects the chances of survival of the business organization, especially early in the life cycle of the business. In essence then, once an investment is made in a partnership it is frozen until agreement can be reached on its withdrawal or on transfer of partnership interests. An example: If Dr. Gibson and Dr. Hernandez are both general partners, Dr. Gibson cannot, one Monday morning after a bad weekend, decide to move down to Florida and to pull out his partnership capital. There will have to be an agreement between Dr. Gibson and Dr. Hernandez about how any capital can be withdrawn or how Dr. Gibson's interest in the partnership can be sold to a new partner. Assuredly, Dr. Hernandez will have a veto right on the potential new partner.

In most states, partnership law requires the dissolution of the partnership upon the death of a partner. The surviving partner (or partners) becomes a "liquidating trustee," whose sole purpose is to wind down the business in the most expedient and economically sound manner. Because of this legal quirk, it is a good idea to arrive at a buy-sell agreement (written separately or as part of the partnership agreement) at the inception of the business. If written correctly, the buy-sell agreement binds both the surviving partner(s) and the heir(s) to a set of actions. In addition, the buy-sell agreement should address the question of how the partners can split or, alternatively, how a partner can sell his or her interest in the business. This sort of decision is made more easily at the beginning of the relationship than when circumstances force it. It is not unusual for partners to show up in court to tell the judge they cannot agree on how to split the business; in fact, they might add, they cannot even agree on what their original handshake agreement covered.

When writing a buy-sell agreement, funding arrangements need to be decided and implemented. It is important to keep the valuation of the business and the funding vehicles up to date. Normally, agreements require funding for the possibilities of retirement, disability, and death. An advantage of a tightly written and correctly executed buy-sell agreement is that everybody, including the taxing authorities, has to accept it. If the business is successful and the partners stay together until one dies, a buy-sell agreement may make a tremendous difference in taxes to be paid as a result of that death.

As a final thought, we have to express our general dislike of partnerships in the health-care field. We would *not* participate in one, due to the difficulty of avoiding liability for our partners' malpractice judgment. Of course we strongly recommend purchasing adequate (read: limits above $1 million) malpractice insurance; however, it is possible that judgments may exceed the insurance coverage. In a partnership arrangement each partner is fully liable for the business liabilities. If our partnership is judged, somehow, culpable and must satisfy part or all of the judgment, then our personal assets may be pursued. This we find unacceptable, especially if it is the situation only because we are the partner of the malfeasant one. While we realize that we cannot escape culpability for our own malfeasance, we do not like to have to pay for the other guy's malfeasance. Since there is an easy way of avoiding this situation (incorporate any time there is more then one doctor in "the house") we would take that route each time.

We can chart the advantages and disadvantages of the partnership form of business:

Advantages
- Relative ease of starting
- Larger supply of capital

- Broader management base
- Sole proprietor taxation
- Potential incentive for employees
- Few regulations

Disadvantages
- Unlimited liability (financial and legal)
- Frozen investment (others have a say over its availability)
- Divided authority
- Lack of continuity

Corporation

A corporation is a separate legal entity with a legal life of its own, independent of the actual owners, the stockholders.

Without following legal citation standards, let's allow the Supreme Court to speak: "A corporation is an artificial being, invisible, intangible, and existing only in contemplation of the laws." In very nice words, it says exactly what is commonly known. The statement, "The company has decided to . . ." is frequently heard, yet corporations do not make decisions. We cannot touch or hold a company. The corporation is clearly intangible. Its decisions are made by people employed by the corporation.

As a separate legal entity, the corporation can exist without the person of the "owner." A corporation owner owns only a piece of paper (stock) which gives certain rights to the owner of that paper. Ownership in a corporation is completely separated from the management of the corporation. It is through the right of the stockholder to vote for members of the board of directors (the ultimate management authority) that a stockholder can influence a corporation's management.

The laws in all states are quite specific in what stockholders can and cannot do. Most of the legal protection exists for the benefit of those stockholders who own only a small part of the corporation. These stockholders are referred to a minority holders. Minority rights may be abridged or eliminated only with the approval of the board of directors and the stockholders. The rights of a stockholder are:

- The right to vote for members of the board of directors and for any issues the board of directors places in front of the stockholders' meeting

- The right not to have stock ownership interest diluted
- The right to share in the profits of the corporation
- The right to share in the liquidation value of the corporation
- The right to transfer stock to others
- The right to inspect the books of the corporation during normal business hours

Currently, most corporate stock is "nonassessable," meaning that the amount paid for the stock at original issue is all that can ever be required to be paid for the ownership rights. Formerly, assessable stock did exist and caused problems in certain situations, frequently after the original owner of the stock had sold it. For example, the new owner (maybe not as keenly aware of the terms of ownership) would receive notification to deposit a sum of money in a corporate account in order for the corporation to be able to continue business or, in bankruptcy situations, to satisfy the debts of the company. No one would be happy receiving such a call unexpectedly.

The concept of the "corporate veil" is an important one: *All actions of the corporation must be authorized actions.* If an officer takes an action which is not authorized, then the officer may be personally liable for the transaction. Professionals decide to incorporate the business to obtain some legal protection from their own and their employees' actions. The corporate veil exist only as long as the corporation is a legal entity. Board and stockholder meetings must be held at prescribed times, and minutes of these meetings must be entered in the corporate record book. Therefore, many owners who are also directors and officers of a closely held corporation will draft minutes (even if they have to meet with themselves) of board of directors' meetings for special high-impact decisions, specifically authorizing the action to be taken. This avoids the piercing of the corporate veil.

Starting a corporation is not all that complex. In reality it works like this: Upon proper application, the state will issue a charter of incorporation to one or more incorporators. The application must include identification of the incorporator(s), the proposed name of the corporation, and the purpose of the corporation. Once the office of the secretary of state has issued the charter, the sale of stock and the start of business activity as specified in the application are permitted. The first order of business is the election of a board of directors and the adoption of by-laws; no corporation can exist without the two. States vary on requirements: some allow a board to exist with one member; some require more. The board's first function is to elect officers of the corporation, those individuals who are actually managing the business. Again, states vary in requirements, some requiring certain offices to be occupied by different individuals, others allowing one person to fulfill all functions. All states require the following positions to be filled: president, treasurer, secretary. Some require a vice president as well.

The process described here applies whether a business is chartered as a general business corporation or as a professional corporation or association. Professional corporation laws, or the state chiropractic association, determine whether a practitioner may form a general business corporation or must apply under the professional corporation rules. The major difference between the two sets of laws is that professional corporation law allows only properly licensed individuals as shareholders of the professional corporation. While the differences between operating a professional or a general business corporation are minimal, the authors favor the latter because of its increased flexibility. Our basic attitude is that since we know reality will force change on us in the future, let's be in the most flexible position possible while still being able to accomplish the task at hand. Check with your state's secretary of state and with your chiropractic association to determine how you must incorporate.

It is difficult to take advantage of the corporation's theoretical liability limitations in the small-business situation of the typical professional. An example: It is doubtful that a bank will lend money to a corporation without requiring the stockholder's signature as a guarantee that, should the business fail, someone can be forced to repay the debt. We can chart the advantages and disadvantages of this business form:

Advantages (theoretical)
- Limited liability
- Broader management base
- Ease of transfer of ownership
- Continuous; lives on when stockholder dies
- Potential tax advantages
- Easier to raise capital (maybe)

Disadvantages
- Not as easy to start
- Government control and (maybe) regulations (charter, by-laws, board, veil)
- Restricted purpose
- Double taxation?
- Lack of secrecy

There are quite a few students who, when we discuss corporations, already "know" that they have to operate a subchapter S corporation. They believe it is the only approach to operating a practice. What these students typically wish to indicate is that they desire to have all income paid out of the corporation each tax year. Again, we understand the objective, but question whether limiting the flexibility is the appropriate approach. If we operate an Internal Revenue Code (IRC) chapter C corporation (the normal tax treatment for corporations), we can determine at the end of the fiscal year if there is a profit and, if so, whether to pay it out to the shareholder employee. In fact, we have until the day the corporate tax return is due (two and a half months after the end of the fiscal year) to make this determination. We can also determine the timing of the payout to the owner; it can be done in the current or in the next tax year of the owner. This flexibility disappears when we elect the chapter S tax status for the corporation. Electing S forces the profit of the corporation to the individual's tax return (Form 1040 schedule E). There is no choice. Therefore, it is against our stance of desiring maximum flexibility. About the only time we would agree with a chapter S election is if we know there will be a loss in the corporation (highly likely in the first few years of operation) and we have an individual tax return with taxable income which can be used to offset the corporate loss.

In recent years, attorneys, accountants, and financial planners have pushed the "new" idea of the Limited Liability Corporation (LLC) to many young practitioners. The authors feel that, again, there is a "fad" sweeping the country. Being critical thinkers (some would accuse us of being contrarians instead) we wish to understand all the ramifications of a proposed move before we make it. Just because everyone else is doing it, does not in and of itself make it right for us. Therefore, we strongly recommend that, before you accept the advice to incorporate under LLC laws, you fully understand the ramifications and limitations in future flexibility thereof.

6

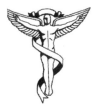 # Office Space

In the United States today, most chiropractors practice in an office away from their home. Though in the past many professionals occupied a home/office combination, only a few of those exist anymore. Only rarely will one find such an arrangement, and then mostly in remote rural areas. As a result, selection and design of a separate office space becomes an issue for most chiropractors. Obviously, in cooperation with spouse and family, a residence will need to be found. The authors feel that most families can handle the latter assignment on their own, but we want to contribute some thought to the office selection.

Location

One of the first decisions that needs to be made, when it is obviously time to own one's own practice, is where to locate. Considerations such as climate, recreational interest, family needs, and lifestyle (city, suburbs, or rural) must be reviewed. Take into account the growth potential of the community. While we find that many students and clients are concerned about the average population per chiropractor, we do not consider this an important factor. As indicated in Chapter 1, we learned from Tom Peters *(Thriving on Chaos: a handbook for a management revolution)* that it is more important to look at the growth potential of the community. We are not market share individuals, we are market growth folks.

Having selected the town, consider the office location. Should it be in a business district? Close to a residential area? If the office is in a rural setting, will it draw from the surrounding communities? Is the town growing or dying? What is the economic base of the community? The larger the commercial base, the better. Research has shown that communities with a young median age are not as interested in health care as those with mid-life or elderly populations. Ethnic communities tend to be more closely knit and may therefore be open only to members of the ethnic group. While the United States, as a whole, is changing in this attitude, it may still be prevalent in certain parts of the country or state.

Choose a location in an area that draws people. Good choices include transition zones between the business district and residential areas, and areas that draw people (for example, shopping centers). The office should be highly visible, easily accessible, with an identifiable landmark close by (for example, post office, well-known store or church), traffic that is not too heavy or fast, adequate parking, and a neat, clean, welcoming appearance. Check with your local community government for handicapped parking regulations. Consider the requirements of the Americans with Disabilities Act (ADA) and the any OSHA (Occupational Safety and Health Administration) requirements which may apply.

When designing your outdoor sign, be sure it has high visibility. Make sure it is illuminated and very professional looking. There are other important considerations, as well:

- Check zoning regulations.
- You should be able to read the sign while moving 30 mph past your office.
- Have it comparable in size to other signs in the area.
- The sign should break the plane of people's vision as they pass by.

Leasing an Office

When leasing office space, have a competent attorney examine the lease before you sign. Any bargaining leverage will only be available before the lease is signed. Use the following questions to guide you in the negotiating process.

- Is the lease figured on dollars per square foot? What will your rent be for one month? For one year?
- If utilities are not provided, what are their estimated monthly costs?

- What services does the landlord provide—heat, electricity, water, air conditioning?
- Will the landlord be responsible for the repair of these services?
- If renovating needs to be done, who will pay for it? (Exterior maintenance is usually the landlord's responsibility.)
- Set up your lease with an option for renewal with first option to buy. With a short lease of one year, try also to include a renewal option with the same terms. The lease should have an option allowing you to *automatically renew*, unless written notice is given to the other party a specified number of days in advance of the renewal date. Some sources recommend a one-year lease. If you have completed your homework on location, this site will be good for you. If you set your lease for four to five years, you are making a major commitment to your practice and will likely work hard to fulfill it. The longer the lease, the more options you have in setting up a lower monthly payment early on, allowing for the lease payment to increase as your practice increases.
- Make sure you are permitted to put up a large sign and that it will be well illuminated. (A contingency of lease approval is that you are allowed appropriate signage.)
- The landlord may require a deposit. Pay it, but insist on a fair agreed-upon interest rate.
- Include a clause giving you the right to remove fixtures you have installed (for example, view boxes, carpet, darkroom plumbing).
- Attempt to have as broad a power to sublease as possible.
- If the building becomes unfit to use (for example, in the case of fire), the lease should be *terminated automatically.*
- The lease agreement should extend and apply to your heir(s), partner, or joint tenant. The lease agreement should automatically transfer to the buy-sell agreement in a partnership. In a cost-sharing proprietorship, the lease should transfer to the other physician(s). For a sole practitioner in a proprietorship, a death-and-disability *"bailout clause"* needs to be written in.
- The landlord should be responsible for the disposal of chemical waste.
- The landlord should pay 100 percent of property taxes and any increase in taxes.

- Any special assessments to the property should be paid by the landlord.
- Review your insurance liability so that it does not cover items already covered by your landlord.
- If you are in a shopping center, get a *"non-compete"* agreement.

The *bailout clause* referred to earlier allows the personal representative of a deceased practitioner to cancel the lease without penalty. This is important for proper liquidation management. The representative ("liquidating trustee" is the term we use in Chapter 5) needs to be able to cut all expenses as soon as possible. This allows collections from accounts receivable to be used for estate purposes. It is extremely important that the sole practitioner carry adequate life insurance. The death benefit will take care of the surviving family's financial needs, and it avoids misplaced concern about keeping the practice open. Unless immediate family members are ready, willing, and able to take over, continuing the practice with substitute physicians does not enhance the value of the practice, but reduces it. Landlords willingly include a death bailout when asked, and will frequently agree to a disability bailout as well.

Owning the Building

Before buying a building or starting construction, know the zoning requirements. Is expansion permitted? It is advisable to have a real estate broker appraise the building for you. This can also be done through your mortgage company. If your building is a home/office combination, this may offer tax advantages. The office portion should have a separate entrance. Your image is important. Don't look as if you're working out of a back room.

Office Design

Deciding on the layout of the office space is the next consideration. It is not necessary or even recommended to start out with a large square footage. Seven- to nine-hundred square feet will provide you with a comfortable and functional working office. Will there be room for expansion? As your practice grows, you will want to adapt your physical structure. The basic office components that you need are reception room, business office, doctor's office/consultation room, x-ray and darkroom, rest room, and adjusting room. Future expansion would include more adjusting rooms, perhaps a dressing room, and a therapy or lab space. Familiarize yourself with your state code for handicapped-access requirements.

The two floor plans shown in figures 5 and 6 are typical of offices designed by starting practices and fall within the recommended space range. A great percentage of professional office spaces offered in the rental market are arranged in either a centralized square or an elongated rectangle. Both designs have advantages and disadvantages.

The advantages of a rectangular design are less build-out required, thus less costly; treatment and consultation rooms are further away from the reception area and thus, even if no sound-deadening material is used, conversations with patients and/or staff are less likely to be overheard; and only two treatment/exam rooms need to be equipped. The disadvantages are the corridor layout may require a lot of movement on the part of the staff; the receptionist will occasionally be great distances from the front when the patients arrive; and treatment/exam rooms double as physical therapy (PT) rooms and thus limit the number of patients that can be seen at a given time.

The square design typically has a little more square footage. As a result, many of the advantages are tied to the extra space: larger waiting room; the assistant/receptionist can stay closer to the front most of the time; separate PT area allows for improved patient flow and scheduling; office gives a more spacious appearance; and rooms can be more "specialized" (for instance, all new patient exams can be scheduled for the room next to the x-ray room). The disadvantages are also mostly tied to the larger square footage: more expensive to move into, and one more room to outfit with tables and diagnostic and physical therapy equipment.

Rarely is an office ready to move into. Most physicians want a number of changes made before they are happy with the layout and appearance. Most landlords take the attitude that such changes are the responsibility of the lessee, however, a little pressure can frequently result in a split of the cost, or the landlord seeing reason and paying for all the leasehold improvements. The longer the space has been unoccupied, the more the landlord will be interested in leasing it. Even without that pressure, reminding the landlord that adding a professional office, such as a chiropractic practice, increases prestige to the property, can often change the attitude about who pays for the build-out or improvements.

When planning the layout, take the time to consider changes that may be required in the future. Most contractors have the incorrect idea

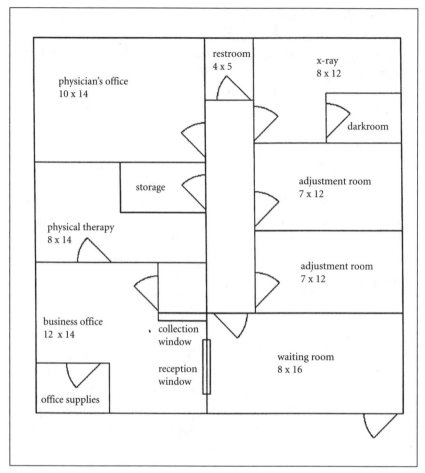

Fig. 6.1. Square office layout with 900 sq. ft. (30' x 30')

that the job must be done the most inexpensive way. As a result they will skimp on electrical and telephone outlets. Insist on an overabundance of those two important items. They are inexpensive to include when the walls are going up, yet rather dear when the electrician has to "fish" them into existing walls. A rule of thumb: you cannot have enough electrical and telephone hookups in a professional office.

When designing or remodeling your office, allow for smooth traffic flow, functional working areas, and a warm, comfortable decor. If you don't have a personal talent for decorating, get the advice of a profes-

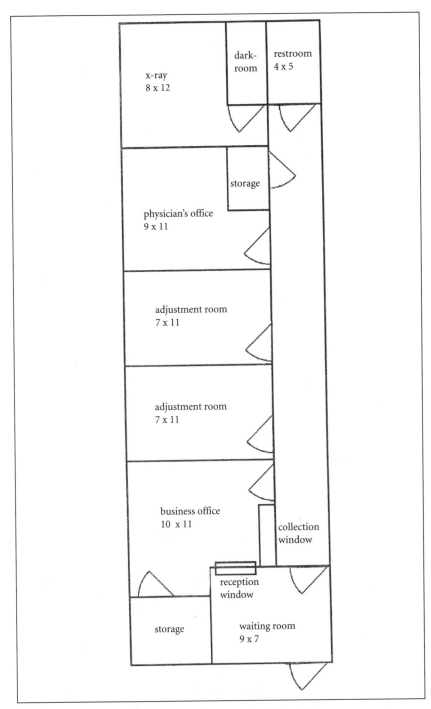

Fig. 6.2. Rectangular office layout with 720 sq. ft. (15' x 48').

sional interior decorator. Many decorators do not charge a fee but rather are paid a commission on the purchases you make. The decorator will help you choose furniture, warm colors, and accessories. Patients' attitudes are affected by their surroundings. A relaxed attitude helps stimulate the healing process. Use plenty of light (indirect is best). Your office is part of your image.

The reception room provides the first impression your patients have of the inner workings of the office and therefore greatly influences their impression of you. The reception room and business office should be adjoining to allow full view from the business office, but allow privacy for telephone calls and business transactions.

Before You Open
There are other tasks that must be addressed before you open:
- Register your license and new address with your state Board of Chiropractic Examiners.
- Obtain county and city licenses to practice, if required; this can be done at the county courthouse and city hall.
- You will need an employer ID number from the IRS. (This is needed as soon as you hire an employee, even your spouse.)
- You will need a state sales tax number if selling supplements and/ or orthopedic supports.
- You will need a Medicare provider number.
- You will need a Medicaid provider number.
- If you become a provider with BC/BS (Blue Cross/Blue Shield), you will need a provider number.
- You will need a permit to take x-rays.
- Contact your post office and get your mailing address.
- Contact the telephone company and get a phone number as soon as possible.
- You will need to have a street address and a telephone number in order to have business cards and letterhead printed. You will need business cards to promote yourself. The letterhead is an important part of promoting your professional image.
- Consider a logo design for your practice. Logos do draw attention to your business name. There are trade logos available and many practitioners utilize them. Generic trade logos identify only the

profession, not the specific practice. In developing individuality for the practice, you might consider having a unique logo designed for your practice. It will ultimately identify your business even without the name.

- Set up a business checking account with your business name and street address.
- Set up a separate personal checking account.
- Prepare to hire at least one part-time person.
- In some states, once you have an employee, you'll need to have worker's compensation insurance. In other states a larger number of employees is needed before the worker's compensation law applies. Check with a local insurance company.
- When you hire an employee, you need to contact the state employment security office for unemployment tax.
- Join your professional societies. Check to see if there is a local society. Do not stand on the sidelines; be a part of the chiropractic community.
- Finalize your personal and professional insurance.
- Finalize equipment purchases and leases.
- Purchase necessary supplies.
- Prepare for opening day and write media notices. Send announcements to local businesspeople (see figure 6.3, next page).
- After you have been open for awhile, set an open house date, prepare media notices, and send announcements to local businesses.

Twenty-four Hour Phone Service

In the beginning, your availability will be vital to your practice. Strongly consider a 24-hour-access service for your patients. Be available for emergency calls. New patients are generated by the doctor who is available after hours for unexpected problems or injuries. Patients can be lost if they have an emergency and you are available only during office hours. Options for a 24-hour phone service are home phone number listed in yellow pages with business number, call forwarding, answering machine (checked routinely), and answering service (checked routinely).

Steven A. White, D.C.
Doctor of Chiropractic

is pleased to announce
the opening of the Whate Chiropractic Clinic
for the practice of Chiropractic

at 321 N. First Ave.
Middletown, Iowa 54321

Office Hours
Mon. to Fri. 8:30 a.m.–6:30 p.m.
Saturdays by appointment

For information or appointment
(319)555-5555

Fig. 6.3. Example of opening announcement.

7

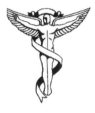 **You Can't Operate Without a Computer**

Any physician browsing through today's professional magazines or walking into any health-care office can easily arrive at the conclusion that no practice can exist without one or more computers. Because the only known research on the subject is totally outdated (1990, Logan College senior research project) or not yet completed (1997, Logan College senior research project), only the powers of personal observation are available to determine penetration of computers into the chiropractic office. The authors are aware of only one practitioner who still operates a practice (and a quite profitable one at that) without a computer in the office. We extrapolate from those observations that most chiropractors use one.

Not Whether, But Which to Buy
The systems offered in the ads vary in cost and power. The choices are bewildering. The non-computer-knowledgeable physician may not know where to start in researching computers, or even what to expect from the instrument. Campuses are full of computer knowledgeable individuals, thus learning the basics is easy and handy for the student. Not so for the practitioner in the field, who now decides to employ this technology. Those individuals often feel at the mercy of a staff or family member, an uncomfortable situation at best, a danger situation at worst.

A physician converting their records from a manual system to a computer-driven system needs to be prepared for potential problems. During this process all manual records are entered in the computer. These are most often the records for the patient accounting system. Conversions can be smooth or fraught with frustration. The way to assure a smooth conversion is to take the time to plan in detail all steps that have to be accomplished.

Today, computer purchasing is like any commodity purchasing. No longer is it necessary, like it was in the seventies and eighties, to be extremely conversant with technology or operating system commands. Buying and operating a computer has become the same process as buying and operating a car. Yet, the bewildering array of options advertised daily in the papers and in specialty catalogs can be confusing and fear inducing to the novice.

The main reason for this confusion appears to be related to two normal human factors. First, many people fear anything having to do with machines whose internal workings are not understood. Yet many physicians drive around in a car daily without knowing a thing about its mechanical functioning. Once it is shown that the operation of a machine can be accomplished without a technician's training, the confusion disappears and the learning starts. The second factor is the failure to recognize the normal learning curve encountered in any exposure to new thoughts, skills, instruments, and processes. Physicians see grade-school children operating computers and think that no learning is involved. It may be advisable for the uninitiated to spend some time at a local high school or community college extension division taking some of the introductory three- and four-night computer courses. The minimum level of knowledge required in the chiropractor's office includes the basic operating system (Windows or Macsoft), wordprocessing, spreadsheet, and simple database knowledge. Patient accounting and other specialty programs for the profession (see list below) probably need to be purchased after some investigation. Few will be available from the local software store. Gathering information at seminars, workshps and from colleagues is the best approach for developing a buying decision.

When in the process of developing the business plan, the entrepreneur takes the time to think about what a computer should be able to do in the office, and a list of repetitive and often tedious tasks can be created:

- Billings, both on-the-spot and monthly
- Ledger and journal entries

- Mailing labels, newsletters, letters (direct mail, recall notices, advertising, etc.), birthday cards, and the like
- Patient file entries
- Insurance claim forms
- Doctor's schedule
- Cash flow and risk analysis
- Narratives, SOAP notes, lab and x-ray interpretations, and the like
- End-of-period accounting functions (end-of-day, -month, -quarter, and -year)
- Practice analyses, which are reports comparing the previous period's financial and office procedures with those of the current period
- Patient clinical histories and other notes

This list makes it clear that a computer may be helpful even at this early stage. Writing loan proposals, marketing plans, direct-mail letters, resumes, and projecting cash flow, can all be completed on a computer.

Software First

The question becomes, What should I buy and what will it cost? The answer is to decide what the computer is expected to do. This will determine the kind of software to be acquired. The software selected will, in turn, determine the hardware to be purchased. Many physicians have thrown away thousands of dollars by not following these steps in order. So repetition is warranted: software first.

Then the hardware choice will be obvious. Hardware may be acquired in stages, as long as the originally acquired equipment allows for expansion. Before proceeding further, some terminology will be helpful:

Hardware: These are all the physical components of a computer, including everything but software.

Software: A set of instructions, written in a machine-readable language, which tells the computer what to do with information provided by the operator or found stored on a disk. Also called a program or application.

CPU/Computer: The Central Processing Unit, typically in boxlike form, which actually does all the work: running the programs, making the calculations, and organizing the information. Common identifications today are 386, 486, 586, and Pentium, whether manufactured by Intel or one of the other chip makers. On the MacIntosh side, most are now equipped with a Motorola manufactured PowerChip.

Monitor: A video screen for communication between the computer and the operator, also referred to as CRT (cathode ray tube) or VDT (video display terminal). Monitors can be color or monochrome. Monochrome monitors show either green or amber.

Printer: Also a communication instrument; provides "hard copy" (printed documents of calculations, letters, or reports generated by the computer).

Modem: An instrument that allows two computers to communicate with each other utilizing either phone lines or direct lines.

Floppy Disk Drive: A slot in the computer that allows for insertion of a diskette and operates not unlike a CD player. It allows the computer to store programs and information to be saved on a floppy disk for later use.

Hard Disk: A storage device the computer uses to store programs and information. Typically a hard disk is installed internally in the computer. It is faster and has a larger capacity than the floppy disk.

Database: A program that stores and manipulates information. In a physician's office, databases are used to record patient addresses for newsletter mailings, birthdates for birthday cards or letters, colleague names and addresses, and so forth. A database holds information the entrepreneur wants to have available quickly. Databases can communicate ("integrate," the programmers call it) with word-processing programs for direct-mail campaigns.

Word Processing: Literally, a program that processes words. It allows for easy manipulation of alpha and numerical information in document form. Narratives, letters, and newsletters can be produced on word-processing programs.

Spreadsheet: A program designed to manipulate figures and perform arithmetical and mathematical calculations. A great tool when preparing cash-flow or risk analysis projections.

Integrated Programs: Programs of different kinds (word processor, database, spreadsheet) that can communicate with each other. Another way to say the same thing: the database and word processor can work together to produce individualized mass-mailing letters.

DOS: Acronym for Disk Operating System. It is a misnomer, because it is a program that operates the entire computer (hardware) system. Originally developed and written by a company called Microsoft, it now has become a generic term as well. The newer computers, such as the IBM PS/2 and its clones, use OS/2 for Operating System Two.

GUI: Graphic User Interface. An operating environment (Microsoft Windows—all versions, and MacSoft) which controls the computer through the use of pictures and symbols on the computer's screen.

Byte: A unit of computer space roughly equal to one letter or character. It is frequently preceded by either kilo- (thousand), mega- (million), or giga- (billion).

Memory: The same concept as the human kind. It comes in two varieties: working memory and storage memory. The working memory indicates the room the computer has for current activity. Normal with most current machines is 8 Mb (8 megabytes or 8,000,000 bytes), although some of the newer, more expensive machines come with 32 Mb (32,000,000 bytes) or more. The storage memory is found on the disks. Normal sizes are 360 K, 720 K, 1.2 Mb, and 1.44 Mb for floppies, and 100 Mb, 800 Mb, or 1, 2, or 3 Gig. Memory can also be said to be:
RAM: Random Access Memory, meaning that the computer can "read" from it or "write" into it, or:
ROM: Read Only Memory, the computer can read it but not write into it.

Speed: As with cars, the concept of computer speed seems to be extremely important to aficionados. It is expressed in megahertz for the technicians. The normal computer user is not especially concerned with the concept until he or she has used the instrument for some time. Initially, everything the computer does, no matter what its speed rating, is done much faster than the operator can think. A good compromise, for the uninitiated, is a computer with 150 to 200 megahertz.

Internet: The general term used to describe the network of computers and services located all over the world encompassing millions of computer users and dozens of information systems including e-mail, Gopher, FTP, and the World Wide Web.

Homepage: The first document that you intend people to see at your location on the World Wide Web.

World Wide Web: An internet service that links multimedia documents together using hypertext. Users can jump between documents using links to view text, graphics, movies, and other media.

Web Browser: A program that allows for easy navigation of the World Wide Web.

While this terminology list is far from complete, it suffices to give the entrepreneur the knowledge required to communicate with computer salespeople. The question now becomes, what software to buy? Most physicians will want to start with a patient-accounting package for insurance and patient billing, a word-processing program, and a database for marketing purposes.

Patient-accounting programs come from cheap to almost unaffordable. The inexpensive ones will keep track of the doctor's daily schedule, the patients, services, and collections. They will prepare patient receipts, patient statements, insurance claims, daysheets, weekly or monthly practice analyses/summaries, and so forth. The cost may be as low as $500. The expensive ones will do all of these functions, and more. Typically, the add-ons are the automatic generation of letters to patients after a certain number of visits, narrative programs, "built-in" word-processing and database functions, and the like. Advertisements show prices to be above $2,500 if the software only is to be purchased, and as high as $10,000 if the hardware is sold in conjunction with it. With the more expensive programs, the main problem seems to arise from the fact that these programs are very powerful and complex. This leads to a steep and long learning curve. As a result, these programs include training sessions for the physician and staff, and thus higher prices. Experience has shown that the inexpensive programs, which come without training, are very user-friendly, and operations can be learned in a few hours.

If one of the inexpensive patient-accounting programs is selected, then the next purchase will be an integrated word-processing and database package. All computer and office supply stores and many appliance and specialty stores have a number of these on the shelf, some for as little as $90–$250. Again, it seems that the less expensive programs are easier to learn to operate. Finally, some inexpensive games and educational programs can be acquired. No one should have to work all the time; occasional relaxation promotes better attention to patients in the long run. Besides, what else can the kids do in the office on Sunday afternoon?

A word of caution needs to be expressed here. As with the increasing complexity and simpler operation of cars, preventative maintenance of computers has become crucial over the recent years. Backing up data files, using programs such as *Scandisk* and *Defrag* (part of the Windows environment) to maintain proper operation of the humongous hard disks, must be done religiously and regularly. Many an entrepreneur does not develop the habit of preventative maintenance of the computer until too late. Once a hard disk crash or other "fatal" error has cost many, many hours and dollars, the habit seems to be developed quickly. It is interesting to note that studies show that most of the major damage to the data, program, and operating files is caused by human reaction to a "fatal" error. In trying to salvage the important information, damage is done to files. Let this be a warning: If you encounter an error and you do not know how to fix it, call the expert (the computer doctor?) and pay for saving your information as well as the needed repairs. It will save time, money, and emotional energy.

Hardware

The hardware to be acquired can be determined from the specified requirements of the software. Normally, a computer with 8 Mb working memory, a 1 or more Gig hard drive, a color monitor, good speed, and a floppy drive, modem, and CD-ROM drive can be bought for between $1,300 and $1,800. Printers are sold separately from the computer. A good medium-speed ink jet printer costs between $200 and $500. Laser printers are becoming more popular and their prices are dropping on a quarterly basis.

The moral of the story is that a physician can have a fine working computer in the office for under $2,000, including all required software. This price is low enough so that if dissatisfaction develops with a part, or all of the system, most physicians can afford to replace it after two or three years. While that is not the recommended attitude with which to buy something, it is an indication of how inexpensive computers have become over the last few years. The work that can be accomplished, even by an inexpensive system, will save many times the purchase price in employee time, printing, mailing label costs, and so forth.

Technology changes are rapid. While there may be a need for current, up-to-date technology for some of the marketing and professional communication work of the practice, the basic patient accounting work can easily be done on an "old" computer. A PC clone with a 386 or 486 processor can frequently be bought at the used computer store for a couple of hundred dollars, including the appropriate dot matrix printer. If a practitioner really has fears and is hesitant to join the computer era, such a machine might be the appropriate tool to acquire to begin the learning process. In addition, for the graduate who has no money but would like to have the benefit of a computer in the office on day one, it could be the route to make that possible.

8

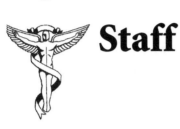 **Staff**

It is rare for a beginning practice to need to employ a full-time assistant; a part-time employee may be all that is needed. In fact, many practitioners start without an assistant at all. Of course, one should be aware of any legal implications of providing health care to members of the opposite sex. For example, it is highly recommended for a male doctor to have a female assistant in the office when giving a female patient an exam. If one starts a practice without an assistant, such appointments can in all likelihood be scheduled at times when a female family member or friend can be present in the office.

The times spent alone in the office are excellent opportunities to become capable with and knowledgeable about the daily business functions of the office. Functions such as patient accounting, bookkeeping, and scheduling need to become ingrained in the business owner's mind. When doctors do not know or understand what needs to be done by the staff, problems often arise. Even when employing a competent, professional staff, the business owner needs to have background knowledge of office operations.

When patient volume has grown to the point that it is appropriate to employ assistants or paraprofessionals, job descriptions for each position need to be created. Other written documents should include employment agreements, detailed skill and personality requirements for each position (for example, the front-desk person needs to be friendly, good with numbers, organized, and a good listener; in addition, an excellent telephone voice is important), vacation and holiday policies, and the like. The best way to develop these documents is to begin with a good, working understanding of the business operation.

Hiring

In preparing to hire an employee, the duties of the position need to be clear to the person doing the hiring. Define and write a job description; include a task list, training and education expectations, performance standards, and desired personality traits. The following outline can be used to develop the description:

Position Description

This is an overall view of the position (includes the position title if appropriate). Include the following items:

- The type of supervision needed in this position (direct, limited, general)
- Supervised by whom? (position and name)
- Nature of work (coordinating of . . . , receptionist, clerical, technician for . . .)
- Level of work (routine, general, administrative, technical)
- Is independent judgment required?
- Is supervision of others required?
- Performs related work as required? (example: "performs other related duties as assigned")
- This should be followed by a specific list of duties and tasks.

Complete job descriptions allow for the easy writing of position advertising. Two examples are:

Receptionist, front desk. Will organize, facilitate, and be responsible for the function of the front desk as listed in the front-desk responsibilities. This position is supervised by the doctor and the person will work in cooperation with all departments.

Billing and insurance/reception. Will organize, facilitate, and be responsible for the functions of billing and collecting from patients and third-party payors. This position provides backup support to the front desk as needed. The position is supervised by the doctor and the person will work in cooperation with all employees of the clinic.

Where to Find Employees

Several options exist for finding employees:
- Checking with patients and their relatives or friends
- Local high schools and community colleges (excellent sources)
- Advertising in newspapers
- Working through an employment agency
- Recommendations by trusted peers
- Applications taken at the desk from walk-ins
- Advertising at paraprofessional schools
- Previous interview sessions

The decision to advertise for the position may depend to a large extent on the time available to fill that position. It is generally a good idea to start the selection process a few months before the position is created or needs to be filled. There will, then, be adequate time to more effectively interview and evaluate the needs of, and the candidates for, the position. Though it is natural to jump at the first candidate who seems to have some of the qualifications, we suggest that a number of candidates be interviewed. This will provide a proper understanding to the interviewer of the possibilities being presented. For some reason, a minimum of three interviews before any hiring decisions are made has always done well for the authors.

Interview Preparation

Once résumés and applications have been collected, interview appointments need to be arranged. Set aside special times for the interviews rather trying to squeeze them in between patients. Within the framework of the interview, the goal is to find the most capable applicant for the position, the one with the best personality and skills, and to communicate accurately and fairly the requirements of the job and the conditions of work to the applicant. Preparation for the interviews will allow one to provide information, and to respond to a candidate's questions on and interest in the following items:

- The specific work performed as part of the job
- The relationship of this function to the rest of the office staff (if any)
- The experience or education required to perform this job
- The nature of supervision the applicant can expect, and the reporting relationships which exist for this position
- The general conditions of work, for example, hours of work, travel requirements, uniform requirements, equipment provided, rotating shifts and/or overtime requirements
- Salary and benefits package provided
- The advancement or promotion potential of this position

Prepare a list of questions to be asked of all applicants; In addition, prepare some questions based on the information available for each applicant before the interview. Job Service of Iowa, in its *Guide to Preemployment Inquiries* (December 1994, publication 70-0006, since updated many times), points out that "it is very difficult for an employer who has included non-job-related questions in an interview to prove that the information generated by such questions was not a part of his or her final decision to hire." While most chiropractic offices are too small (have too few employees) to fall under the federal and most state fair-hiring laws, prudent and sound business practices dictate an open attitude on the part of the interviewer to the possibilities each candidate presents.

The following questions focus on a candidate's experience, education, and relevant personal characteristics, and may be helpful for use in the selection interview.

Questions that address the candidate's previous employment:
- What prompts you to consider leaving your present job?
- What particular parts of past jobs have you enjoyed most? Had the most success with?
- What is your educational background? How have you utilized your education in your past jobs?

Questions that address the candidate's abilities, comfort zone, and availability for this position:
- How comfortable are you working directly with the public, especially if someone becomes upset about some matter?

- What type of supervision do you prefer: close supervision with specific directions or minimal supervision with general directions? Are you more satisfied in a structured job situation or do you like the flexibility to accomplish responsibilities in your own way? What are the personal qualities you see in yourself that lead you to this preference?

Questions that focus on the candidate's self-direction toward goals and self-fulfillment:
- "What the mind can conceive and believe, it can achieve." What does this statement mean to you?
- What are the abilities and/or qualities you see in yourself that you believe will help you to be successful in this position? Where do you think you might have some difficulty?

Close with:
- Is there anything else you would like to ask or discuss, which we have not touched on?

Take a few notes, but listen intently during the interview. This is the opportunity to anticipate the "fit" of the person in the position and the organization. As owner of the practice you will be spending a lot of time in a rather confined area with this person. Can you envision comfort in the relationship which will be established? Are the applicant's attitudes, personality, and behaviors likely to assist the building of the practice? After the interview is completed, take the time to write down impressions and observations which may be helpful during the period of decision making. While all of us feel that our memories are excellent, after two, three, or four interviews, the personalities and skills, as well as specific preferences and dislikes of the candidates, will start to blur. In fact, the authors have found it helpful to "score" the candidate (on a scale of 1 to 5 or 10) as an overall indicator of the "fit"

It is a good idea to keep a list of applicants on file for future reference. This list may generate potential candidates for future openings or may act as a guard against less acceptable applicants who may reapply at a later date. Notes taken during and after the interview will act as reminders for future interviews.

Do not hire after the first interview, instead select a few candidates for a second interview. Sometimes third and fourth interviews should be held. During the followup sessions, it has proven helpful to create a test or trial situation for the candidate to handle. These tests should be as near as possible to the real environment and tasks that will be part of the position. Let each applicant know when the final decision will be made. Send rejection letters immediately to rejected applicants. Thank them for their time and interest and state that you do not see a current fit between the individual and the position.

For professional employees, for instance an associate doctor, it is good practice to have a written employment agreement. The agreement needs to be signed by both parties and should contain all appropriate conditions and requirements. It will become the guideline of employment, requirements of work (hours, dress code), scheduled time off, salary, probation period, and termination specifications. Appendix D contains a sample.

Being an Effective Employer

When hiring staff members, try to hire those individuals with the highest degree of ethics and professionalism. A staff person who is unchallenged is unsatisfied and, thus, frequently unproductive. An excellent way to increase motivation is to improve employees' own estimate of their capabilities. While offering training (both in-house and outside seminars and courses) frequently accomplishes the needed recognition of self-worth, it is smart to occasionally reevaluate the tasks and responsibilities assigned to each individual. If possible (this probably requires more then one employee) job swapping may provide a refreshing outlook and therefore an increase in motivation and quality of work performed. As the practice grows and additional full- or part-time positions are created, use the opportunity to review and redistribute job responsibilities.

For any staff position, the most important responsibility is putting the patient first. The practitioner will need to convey this attitude personally to the staff, through words and action. For example, all staff members should know that patients should not be left unattended for any material length of time, and that they are always to be listened to with real interest and concern. All staff members should be aware that sometimes patients are uncertain whether to tell the doctor about some specific symptom, condition, or occurrence. By informing a staff member, who will pass the information on to the doctor in an appropriate manner, an important communication channel is made available to assist the patient and take care of indicated health conditions.

Office Policy and Management Relations

No matter how many employees a practice has, it is sound business practice to have an office policy manual. Policies provide both management and staff with a common understanding of the way the office should operate. Written communications and expectations are easier to understand than assumptions. In addition, policies provide support for future decisions, and at the same time give the staff security in knowing what is expected of them. If the practice already exists, involving the staff in policy formation will generate a cooperative attitude and may create what the management gurus call "buy-in."

Policies should be followed in all circumstances, and promises should be kept. A quick way to develop distrust, and thus a disincentive to cooperation, is to not perform as promised. This is especially true in the area of compensation. Have paychecks ready on the established pay dates. Make sure there are no mistakes in them. Follow the rules for overtime and vacation pay, and, if necessary provide "comp" time for extra work done and extra time spent. Recognize the effort of each individual, in fact, find a way to compliment each staff member regularly (and meaningfully). Should criticism be necessary, make sure it is provided in a constructive manner and in private.

Employee Incentives

In a study to determine the priorities of employees, the following results were found. They are listed in order of priority as provided by the respondent employees. It is interesting to note that when supervisors were asked their opinion of what employees would list, a different order of priority resulted. Obviously, we listen to the employees:

1. Interesting work
2. Full appreciation of work done
3. Feeling of being included in the decision-making process
4. Job security
5. Reasonable pay

6. Promotion and growth opportunities
7. Good working conditions
8. Loyalty to employees
9. Help with personal problems
10. Tactful discipline

There are many ways incentives and encouragement can be offered to staff. Verbal communication and personal attention and recognition are the easiest and least costly. Therefore, those should be a standard part of the arsenal of everyone with supervisory responsibility. The following list suggests optional incentives. Of course, any incentive should be offered with due regard for and consideration of length of service, job performance, skill level, personal growth displayed, professional licensing, other compensations paid, attitude, habits and skills which promote the practice, and the like.

- Offer to pay for professional license or certification.
- Pay for required CEU's (continuing education unit) to maintain such license or certification. Some seminars may require the staff person to be out of the office, so plan for this eventuality and schedule relief staff if appropriate.
- If seminar attendance is required as part of the employment agreement, pay not only for the seminar, pay the normal wage for work time spent in attending the seminar.
- Pay for X number of sick and/or personal days.
- Regarding paid vacation for employees: Identify in the office policy how many hours must be averaged per week during the year to qualify an employee for paid vacation time.
- Holidays should be compensated for all full-time employees, and an appropriate arrangement needs to be made for part-time staff.
- Profit sharing or year-end bonus programs should be considered.
- Celebrate each staff member's birthday; consider giving part or all of the day off with pay.

Once the practice has been profitable for a number of years, a profit-sharing plan should be considered. In Chapter 18, we look at the financial advantages of such a plan to the owner. In addition to those, there are both psychological and financial advantages to the employees. Profit sharing can maintain or create a positive attitude amongst the employees. It may create a cooperative work climate. Employees are likely to start to feel more involved, and will work to promote the practice. Benefits to be expected from a profit-sharing program include improved employee security, staff involvement and cooperation, and reduction of staff turnover. Profit sharing creates commitment to employees on the part of management, and it acts as a supplement to other employee benefits. Adoption of a plan is a long-term commitment, thus it provides proof of follow-through with promises. Qualified plan regulations require the employer to provide each participant with confirmation of the financial status of the plan and information about the individual's account. Though all these "benefits" exist, the entrepreneur needs to understand that profit sharing is not a substitute for competitive wages and benefits, competent management, and solid personnel practices.

Employee Manual

Employees need support and encouragement from the boss, just as the boss expects to receive them from the employees. Make sure that any input from the owner, which is a prerequisite for the job performance of the employee, is done in a timely and appropriate manner. It would be unfair to blame an employee for not completing assigned work if the entrepreneur was the cause of delay. Help employees with setting goals they wish to accomplish (professional and personal), developing a professional image, supporting the employer, using the schedule book, phone protocol, insurance submission, billing, office procedures, and patient-care related functions. As the practice grows, the staff needs to be able to meet the challenges of a dynamic, progressive practice. By encouraging personal and professional growth, in reality internal promotion of the practice will occur. Improved staff training and skills will result in continued improvement of patient care and education. This, in turn, will increase patient satisfaction. Satisfied patients refer their family, friends, and acquaintances. Amazingly, treating people right is good for business!

Terminating Employees

Terminating an employee is one of the most difficult responsibilities of management. No matter what the reason (cost cutting, underqualification, misconduct, lack of "fit"), written documentation should be created. This documentation needs to include evidence, preferably facts, not opinions, personal judgments, speculations, or assumptions. Having an office policy is, again, an invaluable tool. Discipline policy needs to be part of the employee policy handbook, needs to fairly implemented, and should be progressive: verbal warning, written warning, suspension, and, finally, discharge.

When notifying the employee of the termination it is best to be businesslike. Have complete documentation, present the facts leading to the termination, and state when the termination is effective. Emotions must not be allowed. Do not allow the employee to argue during the termination interview. The decision must be solid and final by the time it is presented to the employee. Depending on the reasons for the dismissal, it is possible to be supportive. If appropriate, offer to provide the employee with a recommendation letter, but make clear that such a letter will be honest and fairly represent the cause and condition of dismissal.

The same laws that govern hiring also govern termination, especially discrimination laws. As stated above, while they may not apply, they make for excellent business practices. In applying discipline, and ultimately termination, the following questions allow for an appropriate review:

- Did the employee fully understand what was expected of him or her? Were the instructions or training adequate and free of ambiguity or contradiction?
- Had the employee been forewarned orally or in writing (manuals, posted rules, written notices) against the kind of conduct for which he or she is being disciplined? Did the employee know of the probable consequences of such conduct?
- Was the rule, order, or standard of conduct reasonable and related to the efficiency and safety of the operations? Was the employee aware of the rule? Can the supervisor prove that the employee knew or should have known of the rule or order?
- In making the decision to invoke the discipline, did management make a full, fair, and objective investigation into the allegations against the employee? Was the employee given an opportunity to be heard and a chance to defend himself or herself before the decision to discipline was made? Were there extenuating circumstances to be considered?
- Was the discipline reasonably consistent with the seriousness of the infraction and generally in accord with the discipline previously imposed on other employees guilty of a similar offense?

- Has the proper consideration been given to the employee's previous record in determining the appropriate discipline? A long-service employee with an unblemished record should be given more consideration than a relatively short-service employee or one whose record has been marginal.

By developing a written policy for employee discipline and termination, common sense, fairness, consistency, and human dignity become part of the management of staff.

Management of Humans

For the success of the practice, a well-run and finely tuned office is a necessity. This does not imply that the people in the office do not have the right to display their humanness. Humor, emotions, care, concern, and empathy are all a part of a well-run office. To develop an efficient team everyone must know his or her responsibilities and see to their accomplishment. But in order to coordinate all of the parts, some kind of management is needed. The manager needs to be well organized, detail oriented, and able to relate to people, yet the overall objectives need to be kept firmly in view. Management must learn to rely on participation rather than intimidation (remember Theory X and Theory Y?). In a small office the doctor is the manager and the supervisor. A doctor should consult with the assistant and the assistant should be part of the appropriate decision making. If the practice is to grow, eventually the owner needs to step down from the supervisor position and function more as a business officer and manager. The day-to-day details may be left to the staff supervisor. In a multi-employee office, one staff person needs to be designated as the office manager. This individual is responsible for the proper operation of the office. The smart entrepreneur, having developed confidence and trust in the manager's abilities, experience, and dedication to his or her philosophy of health care and of business, will not interfere and second guess. Delegation of authority and responsibility is difficult for most owners of closely held businesses, but is indispensable if growth is to continue beyond the point of individual span of control. The business manager needs to be organized and able to work with people. The manager is the decision maker and coordinator of office functions. At the same time the manager needs be capable of appropriate delegation skills, and create a culture, a work environment, that will motivate the employees to provide the best patient care possible. The staff must take an active, responsible role in the business. The doctor, the manager, and staff work together as a team to assure the total quality care of patients. As the team works together, everyone is involved in decision making toward the goals of the office.

In recent years a spate of pamphlets and books has become available to provide the novice supervisor and manager with an understanding of the requirements and desires of today's employees. The authors recommend that it become standard office practice to have a few of these pamphlets in the library, available for each employee who supervises others. Select those which reflect the philosophy and practice of the entrepreneur, then share their concepts. Team dynamics has become a popular topic as well. Again, making the information available will assist in the development of a smoothly cooperating group of individuals. Business gurus are recognizing that a large part of management's task is to provide leadership. Leadership style and culture have, therefore, become common topics in business-related publications. Probably the most important factor in the success of any manager is the capability to think about the effect of any action or decision on the feelings and attitudes of the personnel involved. Take the employee's point of view and analyze the feelings, fears, and concerns the decision or action may present. Frequently, the manager can change the presentation of the action or decision so that those fears are eliminated, and the employee has an opportunity to fully understand all factors which lead to the decision. Communication—effective, honest and open—may well be the secret to developing a supportive and committed staff. Shared vision is a powerful driving force. American business, we are sorry to note, had to experience an extended period of difficulty from a competitive point of view before this message was understood. Today, signs that we have accepted modern human management concepts are all around us. Owners of chiropractic offices need not be behind the times in this respect. The golden rule, simple to understand and easy to implement, is, "Treat people as they wish to be treated".

Part Three

How Do You Open an Office?

9

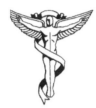 # Associate
or Incubate

In many professions joining a firm is recognized as the final portion of the professional education process. Although lawyers, accountants, and architects do not use the term "associating" as frequently as chiropractors, for many years they have used the concept. Those professions see the purposes of the period of work immediately after professional school as follows: gaining experience and clinical knowledge under the tutelage of an experienced professional; learning how a successful practice is run on a day-to-day basis and from a business point of view; and developing experience in generating and handling clients, working with office staff, and dealing with suppliers. No matter how it is expressed, the period seems to be a short-term relationship, lasting from one to three years, after which the professional is prepared to open a practice from scratch or buys an existing practice or joins a group practice as a full member.

During this phase of professional polishing, most often the young (in experience) professional is an employee. Sometimes, especially among lawyers and accountants, the young professional is an independent contractor. In either relationship, the senior professionals are available for assistance in dealing with the technical, professional, and business affairs of practice. For some reason only rarely do we observe this attitude in the chiropractic profession. While understanding of the concept has increased in the profession over the last decade, too often we still see the Dr. Experienced attitude of wanting to hire "slave labor" and the Dr. New attitude of "I'm only interested in the money." Neither attitude is productive if the objective of the period is to develop mature, capable, practicing chiropractors.

It is difficult for the new graduate to find an associate relationship in chiropractic, because no formal programs of introduction exist as they do in other professions. Recent graduates from chiropractic school are left to their own devices to find willing field doctors who will take in a new associate. Individual negotiations are therefore required, and no real standard of relationship between Dr. Experienced and Dr. New exists. An analysis of what each party is looking for is in order for better understanding.

Dr. New should want the above described experiences and a living wage. It is important that these desires are communicated to Dr. Experienced. Communications should be open, truthful, and detailed during the process, or unrealistic expectations may grow on either side. The term "living wage" will have different meanings depending on the situation, location, and circumstances. Too many new graduates have unrealistic expectations. Dr. Experienced and the chiropractic profession do not owe Dr. New anything. Yet many negotiations do not even get started because Dr. New wants to be paid $4,000 or more per month for hanging around in the clinic. To Dr. Experienced this up front "demand" shows that Dr. New is unaware of some basic facts of business economics. In most instances, to pay such compensation would require that Dr. New produce an additional $100,000 or more in annual collections for the practice. The chances of a brand-new doctor producing that level of revenue in the first year after graduation are, honestly, rather small. The authors have seen only very few practitioners do it.

The chances of establishing a successful relationship are much higher if Dr. New would use the initial few contacts with Dr. Experienced to develop a feel for the opportunity which may exist. He might well ask himself such questions as, Is this the kind of practice I envision myself operating in the future? Are the patients the kind I expect I will draw to my practice? Is the atmosphere of the practice, the interaction of the doctor with the patients and the staff, between the staff and the patients, the kind I want to have in my practice? Is the office layout and location what I would choose? Are the techniques and modalities what I would practice? Is the marketing of the practice comfortable for me? Is the volume of business about what I desire to develop? All those are the more important factors to view in the beginning. In fact, when we counsel practitioners on finding an "associateship," we suggest these questions and advise that the first and second visits should really have a "rule out" purpose. We have come to express it as looking for "red flags." Red flags are observations that require further information from the doctor, the staff, the patients, the community, and so forth. Red flags can be lowered if the additional information provides a satisfactory explanation. Our rule of thumb is: "Three red flags raised and not explained is cause for me to walk away from the 'opportunity.'" It is sometimes hard for students to understand, but finding an appropriate associateship is not a long distance affair. Dr. New needs to visit the practice a few times before deciding whether to continue his interest in pursuing the relationship.

Dr. Experienced has desires regarding the relationship as well. The typical physician willing to take in a new graduate owns a busy practice and may be hoping to spend less time in patient care, to become more of a business manager, and spend the freed-up time to market the practice for further growth. Maybe Dr. Experienced is interested in "slowing down" and wants to turn over some of the workload to a younger individual. Possibly Dr. Experienced is struggling to meet overhead payments and needs assistance with the cash flow, or it could be that she has run out of mental energy and is looking for support and renewed vigor in continuing the difficult life of running a practice. Some field doctors feel the need to retain the upper hand in the relationship with Dr. New. This attitude makes sense in the beginning of the relationship, but should shift over time as confidence is built in the skills of Dr. New.

Dr. Experienced should want to have a few opportunities to visit with the potential Dr. New as well. After all, bringing an additional doctor into a practice can create major upheaval and could possibly have a negative effect on the ability of the practice to continue to draw patients. While it is obvious that such an occurrence would have drastic consequences for Dr. Experienced, we see too many such doctors just interested in hiring someone, almost as if they were happy just to have a warm body present.

Only after both parties have reached the point of comfort with the possible relationship should compensation of Dr. New become a topic of concern. The authors are convinced that professional business relationships should be based on concepts of fairness and equity, and professional ethics. With regard to compensation, this translates to an understanding that in the long run a professional will be "paid" exactly what he is worth, not a penny less and not a penny more. Therefore, the real issue is the initial period of working together: How do we arrange for a living wage for Dr. New while he is trying to learn and get a handle on the profession?

Most often, a detailed, realistic list of expenses Dr. New must pay will allow Dr. Experienced to understand the financial situation, and the negotiators can then arrive at a suitable solution. The term "realistic" has little flexibility in the way we use it here, maybe "minimal" would be a better choice. Many a Dr. New feels that student loans must be paid off as rapidly as possible. While we totally support the concept of becoming debt free as speedily as possible, student loans are the least of the debt problems if managed correctly. Moratoria (periods when no payment is required) are frequently offered by lenders and deferment is built into almost all student loan programs. Deferring the start of student loan payments for a year, eighteen months or two years, will allow Dr. New to live modestly and develop the necessary skills and confidence to generate new patients, office visits, fees for services and collections (the reader should by now be well aware of the progression) adequate to produce a profit big enough to live on and to make student payments. We see young practitioners develop incomes from practice in the $60,000 to $100,000 range in their third year in practice all the time; rarely, though, do we see it in the first year of practice. (Fairness dictates that we acknowledge, as well, knowing chiropractors who never reach those levels.)

Having admonished Dr. New, we need to do the same for Dr. Experienced. We have seen situations where the established professional wishes to keep total control of the new one's development. Sometimes, she will try to accomplish this by offering low compensation and requiring unreasonable time and attention from the recent graduate. In addition, she will confuse the issues of employment and independent contractor status. The confusion stems from the desire to remain the physician in charge and the potentially conflicting desire to avoid payroll tax and malpractice liability. Once such physicians realize that the ownership of the practice assures that they remain in charge, and that payroll and malpractice costs can be viewed as part of the total compensation package, negotiations can proceed on a more reasonable level and yield a workable agreement. Dr. Experienced should keep in mind that the profession and the patients have been quite kind and rewarding to her. Providing an opportunity and assisting new blood to enter the profession is rewarding work in and of itself. It is the right—the professional—thing to do. It assures that chiropractic will grow and improve in service to mankind.

The best result of the process of negotiations is what the authors refer to as an incubator agreement. As in other industries, incubators exist to help new businesses form and survive the dangerous period referred to as the Valley of Death. Many states, municipalities, and large business organizations realize that economic growth can occur only if new businesses are started and manage to grow and avoid bankruptcy. These entities will create, at a specific location, an organization that provides inexpensive rental, clerical support, office equipment, management support, and marketing know-how. The incubator agreement tries to imitate this structure. Its main purpose is to allow Dr. New to start a practice without financially damaging the existing clinic. The end results are stronger chiropractic businesses and a better profession. Whether the incubator period leads to continued cooperation between Dr. Experienced and Dr. New (for instance, a partnership, a corporation with two owners, or continued cost sharing) or to a split and the creation of two office locations, the purpose of the agreement has been accomplished.

A short review of the possibilities of the two legal relationships is necessary.

Associating as an Independent Contractor

Initially, the concept of an independent contractor relationships may be uncomfortable for both parties. Dr. Experienced is concerned that there will not be enough control. Dr. New wants guarantees. Both expectations are unrealistic, not available in real life. We have started asking Dr. New the question, "What can be more of a guarantee than to depend on your own skills and determination?" Of course self confidence and realism are required to answer the question as intended. As an independent contractor, Dr. New is starting a practice from scratch in the office space of, and with the equipment, belonging to, Dr. Experienced. Compensation should flow from Dr. New to Dr. Experienced. It should be adequate to cover the use of space, equipment and other services provided. The authors favor a flat monthly payment. The amount can rather easily be negotiated by looking at the cost of what Dr. Experienced will provide Dr. New. Payment of the compensation should be made on an agreed-upon date each month and late payment fees and penalties should be included in the agreement. We do not favor the rather common concept of compensation being a portion of collections of Dr. New. This approach has built-in dissatisfiers for both parties. In the beginning, Dr. Experienced is likely to receive less than what was expected because Dr. New is not developing the practice as fast as was anticipated. Later in the relationship, Dr. New will become dissatisfied with paying more (sometimes much more) than it would cost to operate a separate office. We have observed that most often both parties walk away from the concept of a flat monthly payment because of a concern about Dr. New's capabilities of making the financial commitment. We feel that the solution to this concern is the borrowing of necessary funds. Dr. Experienced can introduce Dr. New to the banker, or Dr. New can borrow from family or friends, or Dr. Experienced can act as banker for Dr. New. Appendix E (Sample Agreement One) shows that this is a viable approach.

We tend to shy away from relationships which include an expectation that the staff of Dr. Experienced will support Dr. New as well. In chapter 8 we made our attitude clear: at the start, for cost control and education purposes, Dr. New should operate the business completely. In addition, Dr. Experienced's employees are loyal and supportive to him; it may be unfair, and probably will be ineffective, to ask them to split that loyalty. It rarely works in real-life situations. It needs to be realized that in operating a practice of one's own, all costs need to be paid for. Therefore, besides the cost of the space and the equipment, the independent contractor will need to budget for advertising, mailing, insurance, education costs, and the like.

Finally, it should be noted that a non-compete clause has no place in an independent contractor's agreement. After all, the objective of the contract is to start a new practice in the established location. If that is not competition, then what is?

Associating as an Employee

The employer-employee relationship is well known to most Americans. The employer makes all decisions regarding the work to be performed by

the employee. Who is to be treated, when, where, and how are all decisions in the purview of the employer. The employee is compensated on a
wage or salary basis and all payments received from the patients and third-
party payors belong to the employer. A smart employer will reach an
employment agreement with a professional that incorporates the concepts established earlier with regard to the value of the professional employee. Base salary is normally paid, and bonuses based on production
should be included. Both parties need to be realistic in this regard: the
employer has costs directly related to the amount of compensation paid
(see Chapter 14 for payroll taxes) and should have the advantage of making a profit on the work of the employee. The professional employee should
realize that the moneys received in the form of a paycheck are not the
only compensation received from the employing practice. Frequently benefits such as insurance, vacation and holiday pay, continued education
expenses, mileage reimbursement, and others are also received. Were the
employee self employed, those costs would be paid out of collections before profit can be paid to the entrepreneur. A similar thought process
needs to take place in case of an employment agreement. Non-compete
clauses are common and belong in an employer-employee relationship.
The sample employment contract in Appendix D may give both parties
some further guidance.

Final Thoughts on Professional Cooperation

As Hamlet might have said, "Whether to associate or incubate, that is the
question." Well, maybe that is a slightly more liberal translation than appropriate, but at least it makes the point that chiropractors, recent graduates as well as established practitioners, have decisions to make that are for
both personal and professional benefit. Weighing the factors involved is a
time-consuming and difficult affair. This, all the more so, because egos
and emotions are involved. Individual decisions, made many times in many
places, leading to many relationships, will determine whether the
chiropractic profession will grow and develop commensurate with the opportunities presented by the health-care consuming public. Established
professionals in other fields have long realized that the days of the single
practitioner are gone. Few physicians can any longer carry the financial
and mental burdens of rising rental costs, increasing staff demands, and
more stringent and detailed requirements of insurance companies and

governments. Thus, they opt for group practices. Chiropractic is still very much a "loner" kind of profession. The authors feel that there is a benefit to looking at the experience of others and learning lessons from it.

The Option Not Separately Mentioned: Starting from Scratch

There are some individuals who graduate from chiropractic school who, because of prior experience, personality, or maybe just "because," should consider opening their own office immediately. These new doctors do not need seasoning and have adequate self-confidence and skill to operate a practice once they are properly licensed. While the preceding paragraph displays our attitude toward solo practitioners, there are individuals, places, and times where they make sense. Though we do not have a specific chapter addressing the issues involved in starting from scratch, we feel that we will adequately assist those individuals by means of all the material in this book. Really, the differences in starting from scratch, incubating, or buying a practice occur in the beginning few months. We trust that the specific examples, in the appendices and elsewhere, are of adequate assistance to those considering such a move.

10

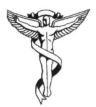 **Buying a Practice**

For the individual fresh out of school, buying an existing practice may be an excellent way to start professional life. In addition, there may come a time in the life of the entrepreneur with an existing practice when there is an opportunity to purchase a second practice from a colleague. Thus, a discussion of the topic is required.

All That Goodwill Just Sitting There

An existing practice offers the potential of a shorter, shallower Valley of Death than does starting from scratch. The location, patients, equipment, and so forth, already exist. As a result, the office should be easier to operate and to run smoothly, compared to a new business. The purchase of a practice normally avoids most or all of the negative cash flow that is unavoidable in a "from scratch" operation, and bankers will be more likely to display a positive attitude because the banker can review the operation's success over the past few years and develop a track record of profitability. This, in turn, allows for more confidence in the projections. If nothing else, the expense factors are already known.

Just because a practice has patients and generates an income for the current owner is not a guarantee of success for the new owner. Because the current owner is likely to expect some or all of the sale price in cash up front, investigation, analysis, and plan development may be even more important than when starting a new business. The old saw, Buyer beware, definitely applies; many a young physician has been sold an empty bag!

What Needs to be Considered

When buying a practice, many variables will need to be considered, including location, accessibility, parking, patient socioeconomic levels, community growth potential, and office remodeling needs. In addition, it must be determined why the practice is for sale, whether there is life remaining in the practice, or whether it is stagnant and will need an impossible amount of energy to regenerate. Concerns such as whether the buyer's and seller's treatment techniques, method of practice, and the like are compatible ought to be addressed. An initial list of questions to ask will look very similar to the list created for Dr. New in the previous chapter for the first few visits. In fact, the "red flag" approach works well here too. In addition, other questions may arise: Will you retain the existing equipment, or will you have to buy or lease new equipment? Are there any liens on the property or the equipment? A complete inventory of the business will need to be created. Practice statistics and tax returns for the last few years should be reviewed, and a determination of the sources of new patients may be crucial. If the building is owned by the current practitioner, will the purchaser have an opportunity to buy it, either now or in the future after renting it for a period of time? In either case, appraisals of the land and building will be required. The equipment should be appraised at market value. Chiropractic equipment distributors or x-ray dealers are capable of performing the appraisal and frequently will do so for minimal fees. It is wise to have an accountant involved in some stages of investigation and in the development of some of the cash-flow projections and pro forma financial statements. Need it be mentioned that before any contract is signed, an appropriate attorney should review it?

Some people feel that by starting discussions with Dr. Experienced they are committing to the purchase of the practice before they have adequate knowledge to make the decision. Nothing could be more incorrect. Stating to Dr. Experienced, "I'm interested in discussing the purchase of your business," does not make it a done deal. There is nothing wrong with proceeding with the negotiations only to come to the realization that actual purchase would not be in the best interest of the budding entrepreneur. The moment one realizes this is the moment to communicate it honestly to the seller. Most owners of existing businesses are interested in a transaction that is worthwhile for both sides. They have pride in the work previously accomplished, and will express it as a desire to see their patients properly cared for. If the deal is right, both the seller and the buyer are completely satisfied and happy, even many years after the transaction. The desired outcome is a win-win-win for the seller, the buyer, and the patients.

Making the Transition

Smart business sense tells us that making any changes in a practice may lead to a loss of patients. From the patients' point of view the practice belongs as much to them as it does to the doctor. Patients become used to being treated a certain way, having the office look just so, and seeing the same staff members each time they come in. Changing doctors, with whom the patient has a very personal relationship, is hard enough to adjust to. Making other changes at the same time is therefore not advisable. Any changes that the new owner wishes to make should be made slowly and one at a time. It is especially important to keep the same fee schedule for a reasonable period, say half a year to nine months. Keep in mind why a practice purchase is being considered in the first place: it offers the possibility of getting into practice by having an established cash flow. If patients leave to go to their second favorite doctor instead of the purchaser, cash flow will drop. This would defeat the original intent of the practice purchase transaction. Assistance of the selling practitioner during the takeover period is crucial. Many fine discussions of the concepts of this cooperation exist in chiropractic literature, therefore, we do not need to specifically address it. Keeping some or all of the staff may be advisable, at least for a period. It is a double-edged sword, however. While the staff can assist Dr. New in cementing relationships with the patients, it is also possible that the staff may steer patients away. This sometimes happens inadvertently, especially if there is a personality conflict between Dr. New and the staff member. Frequently such a conflict is nobody's fault—Dr. New just does not do things the way Dr. Experienced did them.

Types of Patients in the Purchased Practice

Earlier, mention was made of the importance of knowing the sources of new patients for a practice. The main reason for the emphasis is that it is important to determine if the source will continue to generate patients for the new owner. By way of example, a large portion of personal injury (PI) patients would decrease the value of the patient files to the purchaser. Reasons for this attitude include the fact that attorneys most often generate those patients and that the doctor-attorney relationship in all likelihood will not transfer (just as the patient always has a second favorite health-care provider in mind, so also the attorney has a second favorite doctor in mind for referral). Also, most PI patients are of an allopathic attitude (symptomatic relief is all I want) with a situational reason for coming in for treatment in the first place. Rarely do PI patients refer others to the office. PI is not the only source of patients which may not transfer. Almost any specialty group (sports injuries, pediatrics, geriatrics, Boy Scouts, and other such personal relationship sources of patients) will only continue to be a source of patients if Dr. New is also a member of the group. Frequently, sources of the personal interest kind are not the same for the seller and the buyer. It will take some time before Dr. New has become enough a part of the community that his personal sources can replace the volume of new patients Dr. Experienced generated from his sources.

What Is Being Purchased?

There are at least two ways of thinking about the purchase of a practice. One is to assume that the entity, the whole practice, is being acquired. The other approach assumes that only some of the assets of the practice are being obtained. Each approach has advantages and disadvantages. Acquiring the entity allows the purchaser to continue to operate as if nothing has happened and therefore has the advantage that the consuming public sees little difference other than the new doctor. The disadvantage of this approach (at least lawyers tell us so) is that liabilities are also acquired. Thus, if in the future some long-standing but undiscovered debt of the practice surfaces, the new owner may be forced to satisfy the debt. The advantage of an asset purchase is that only the specifically named items will transfer in ownership. Typically, three assets are acquired: space, equipment, and patient files. The disadvantage of an asset purchase deal is mostly to the seller; the remaining assets may need to be liquidated or disposed of in other ways.

The Asset Purchase Approach

The three assets to be acquired can be valued separately. Starting with space, there are two possibilities: either the seller owns the property or it is a leased space. In the latter case, most office leases require the buyer to negotiate directly with the landlord for a new lease. Sometimes this can be as simple as agreeing to take over the existing agreement; sometimes a whole new lease with new rental amounts and periods needs to be hammered out. Rarely does the practice owner deserve any compensation for space in the case of an unexpired lease. If the current practitioner owns the building, as stated earlier, it is most often best for both sides to have him continue to do so for a period of a few years. The advantage to the property owner is that renting the building will generate monthly income (in reality, the property-owning chiropractor changes business endeavors, from chiropractor to landlord), while maintaining a valuable asset. Should the new chiropractor not succeed, or should she wish to move the practice to another location, at least the landlord has sellable property. In this situation, most office rental agreements we have seen include a first right of refusal clause. This instrument forces the landlord to offer the sale of the office building to the chiropractor who purchased the practice. Normally a three- to five-year period is provided for. This allows the new doctor to establish herself and to generate the needed cash down payment for the building.

Purchasing the equipment (and supplies) of the practice is also rather easy. As indicated above, there are a number of distributors who will gladly provide a market-value estimate in return for a small fee. Three levels of estimate, and therefore fees, exist. The lowest is the opinion: the distributor walks through the office, takes a few notes, and then provides a letter stating an opinion of the total market value of the equipment. The second is more precise. After taking inventory of the equipment the distributor supplies a report which details the price at which the same or similar piece sold within the recent past. The third approach, and the hardest to convince the distributor to offer, is what we call the guaranteed market value assessment. It is basically the same as the last approach but now the letter contains a statement indicating a readiness by the distributor to purchase the equipment from the rightful owner at the listed value, at the option of the owner, within a rather short (typically three months) period in the future.

The hardest asset to value is the patient files to be purchased. No one really will know the value of these files until sometime in the future, after Dr. New has operated the practice for a long enough period of time to develop a stable profit level. At such a time, a net present value calculation could easily determine the hindsight value of the asset. Few sellers are interested in waiting the three to five years required to agree to the value of the patient files. In counseling purchasers, therefore, we advise taking the cash-flow valuation approach. It is an agreement that the buyer will pay the seller a portion of the collections from the purchased patient files for a stated period of time. One- or two-year periods are commonly agreed upon. Forty to fifty percent is the most common proportion we see. Occasionally, Dr. Experienced will object to this approach, expressing fear that Dr. New will not work the files "hard" enough. While this would be totally opposite to the purchaser's interest, it is an emotional reaction by the seller. Frequently, in those cases, a compromise is reached that the cash flow will continue beyond the original period if a stated amount has not been paid. In the extended period then, a smaller portion (typically half the original proportion) of collections is turned over to the seller. In any case, once the stated amount is paid, or the extended period has run out, payments will stop. The reader may feel this approach to be cumbersome. In reality, it is how almost all businesses are bought and sold, based on the cash flow expected to be generated to the new owner of the business. With today's computerized patient accounting programs, the record keeping is very simple. The purchased patient files are assigned to a separate provider number, the monthly reconciliation or practice analysis for that provider number is then printed, and the appropriate portion of the collections is paid to the seller. Sometimes the issue of referrals from the purchased patient files will become a point of discussion. Dr. Experienced feels that those referrals need to be compensated for. We disagree. Had Dr. Experienced continued to operate the practice the referrals would belong to him, now that Dr. New operates the practice the referrals came as a result of the patients' satisfaction with her work.

The Entity Purchase Approach

When buying the entity of the practice, most often a large portion of the purchase price is paid up front. The hard part of this, even if the purchaser has the financial capacity to do so, is to determine the appropriate value of the practice. Other professions have generated some rules of thumb. For instance, in the insurance industry, it is common practice to sell an agency for one time the annual commissions earned plus the value of any office furniture, fixtures, and equipment. In reality this approach is possible for any business. Commissions earned in the insurance industry equate to collections in the chiropractic profession. The major difference is that chiropractic office collections are much more volatile than insurance agency commissions. Therefore, the multiplier may need to be adjusted downward to reflect that uncertainty. We have been involved in successful practice transfers using this approach and have used somewhere between 40 and 60 percent of collections as a base for the price. A different approach we have used successfully is to calculate the expected first-year profit from the practice for Dr. New and to use it as a basis. Clearly, cooperation between purchaser and seller is necessary. It needs to be stated that mandatory pieces of information for the purchaser are the last three years of business tax returns for the practice. Without this historical information a solid basis for projection of collections or profit does not exist.

As a general rule, buying accounts receivable should be avoided for the benefit of both Dr. New and Dr. Experienced. Patients feel they owe Dr. Experienced for services rendered. If Dr. Experienced "disappears," few patients feel any compulsion to continue making payments to Dr. New. Therefore, Dr. New cannot benefit as much as can Dr. Experienced from existing accounts receivable. Besides, Dr. New rarely has the cash to pay up front for future uncertain cash flow. In some situations it is appropriate for Dr. New to act as a receiving agent for Dr. Experienced. If, for instance, Dr. Experienced leaves for extended travel shortly after selling the practice, and Dr. New continues one of Dr. Experienced's long-time staff members in the employment, collection of accounts receivable by the practice may be effective. In this situation, Dr. New is normally rewarded with a percentage of collections as compensation for the efforts of the practice. This compensation is deducted from collections before Dr. Experienced is paid.

In the highly unusual case that accounts receivable are purchased by Dr. New, careful review and valuation is required. Complete access to the books, patient ledgers, and account histories is imperative. A good, solid practice might have accounts receivable of three times the month's gross services. If accounts receivable are greater than this, the collection policy may have been implemented too liberally or there may be a large amount of personal injury receivables. If the practice accepts insurance assignment and has a large number of verified claims outstanding, a relatively high percentage can be paid for such accounts. Cash accounts are harder to collect. The lower the percentage paid for these, the better. Take into consideration the age of the accounts. A graded schedule of value of accounts, based on age, may be appropriate. A safety valve is to return uncollected accounts receivable to the selling doctor after a set period of time. Of course all this needs to be included in the purchase agreement. In addition, a letter, signed by the selling doctor, stating that all checks can be deposited into the new owner's account and giving permission to contact patients, attorneys, and insurance carriers should be obtained.

Many doctors will want to sell the practice's goodwill. When asking for this, they think of location and patients' confidence. It is advisable to consider that these values are included in the patient files purchase amount, or, alternatively, to include the goodwill value in a non-compete agreement. Non-compete agreements state that the selling doctor agrees not to practice chiropractic for X number of years, within Y number of miles. This non-compete agreement is amortizable (i.e., tax deductible) more rapidly then goodwill. For an example of treating goodwill, see the case study later in this chapter.

Make sure there is a list of all equipment, supplies, and inventory, including model, color, and serial numbers. Inspect all leases or mortgages. The purchase of the equipment can be outright or, if need be, it can be bought and then sold to a leasing company under a leaseback provision. It is important that the equipment be in good mechanical condition. If necessary, assuming the equipment is mechanically good, it can be refurbished for a rather low cash outlay. The investment is much less than that of purchasing new equipment.

A Case Study

While the following case occurred some ten years ago, the authors feel it still has value as a description of the process of purchasing a practice. In addition, Appendix H presents a business plan and loan proposal for a practice purchase. The names and location have been altered in the following examples, but the structure and purpose of the transaction have been left unchanged.

Dr. Jeffrey Jones has been operating the South Side Clinic on a part-time basis since 1978, when he purchased the office from his predecessor. Initially, the practice was a busy one, but over the years Dr. Jones has reduced the patient visit count because he teaches at a local college. He is in his mid-forties, and his responsibilities at the school have increased over the years. His time and energy commitment to the practice have decreased as a result. Approximately ten years ago Dr. Jones was married, and he now has two daughters, ages five and three. He wants to spend more time with his family, and he is selling this practice to create that time.

Dr. Jones and his family live comfortably on his college income and the part-time income from his wife's job. The practice has operated for the last three years with approximately $30,000 in collections and a taxable profit of $21,000. Dr. Jones has realized for a few years that he is underutilizing his facilities and has allowed Dr. Davis to use the office on a part-time basis. The two doctors are never in the office at the same time, and have a financial arrangement such that Dr. Davis pays Dr. Jones a flat $1,000 per month for use of the facilities. Initially, this arrangement worked well, but over the last year and a half Dr. Davis has skipped two or three monthly payments. Dr. Jones is not interested in trying to collect these missed payments. The agreement between the physicians is a hand-shake agreement.

Dr. Mayfair and Dr. Choo graduated a semester apart in 1988 from the nearby chiropractic school. They have been looking for an opportunity to buy a practice and are introduced to Dr. Jones by a mutual acquaintance. Neither of the new doctors has any prior business experience, and they feel uncertain about how to proceed. Both have large student-debt obligations, and neither has any money worth mentioning. They have tried on a few occasions to obtain bank financing to start a practice from scratch, but the bankers seem concerned about the existing financial situation of both physicians.

The mutual acquaintance suggests that they might want to look at the practice as a "starter" package. Analysis of the financial information shows that the overhead is covered even if two-thirds of Dr. Jones's patients do not stay with the new owners. The following agreement results from negotiations:

Ownership Transfer Agreement

This agreement, signed this 30th of January, 1989, by and between Jeffrey Y. Jones, D.C., herein after referred to as "seller," and an entity consisting of Sherri Mayfair, D.C., and Susan Choo, D.C., hereinafter referred to as "purchaser," is made to transfer ownership of South Side Clinic from seller to purchaser. Purchaser intends to be a corporation chartered by the State of Missouri, and the intent of this document is to recognize such business form, once chartered.

Seller agrees to sell to purchaser the chiropractic practice known as South Side Clinic, free from any encumbrances or debts. The practice, for purposes of this agreement, is more precisely defined as: the practice name, certain patient lists, patient chiropractic files and records, furniture, fixtures, office equipment, personal computer together with the installed software, chiropractic equipment, instruments, supplies, a lease for the occupied office space, certain security deposits with the landlord and possibly with certain utility companies, and leasehold improvements, all located at 512 South Boulevard, Suite #1, in Canada, Missouri.

Seller agrees to assist purchaser in obtaining transfer of said lease to purchaser on the records of the landlord, South Center Corporation. Seller agrees, if this turns out to be the only lease transfer approach available, to remain a party to the lease until its expiry on July 31, 1991. Seller has informed purchaser that the Simplified Physicians Accounting software may be subject to a transfer-of-ownership fee. If so, this transfer fee will be the responsibility of purchaser, should they decide to use the program.

Purchaser agrees that seller has provided full disclosure of all pertinent facts involved in the sale of this practice, and purchaser warrants that they are aware of the constituting factors of a chiropractic practice, and have done the requisite information gathering about the practice to make an informed purchase decision. Purchaser further warrants that seller has not made any promises as to the revenue purchaser may be able to obtain from this practice. Seller has disclosed Schedule C of his 1986 and 1987 tax returns and a preliminary Schedule C which he intends to file with his 1988 tax return (seller reserves the right to make changes in this Schedule C if he so desires. Any such change shall have no effect on this agreement). Seller has further provided purchaser with information about the patients new to the practice, the number of x-rays taken, and the total charges for services, all for the calendar year of 1988. All parts of the practice and the practice as a whole are sold on an "as is" basis.

Seller has informed purchaser that he has for a period of time allowed Demetrius Davis, D.C., to use South Side Clinic's facilities for Davis's proprietorship practice at stated monthly charge. Purchaser recognizes that seller has no power to make any agreement for Davis, and that they will have to reach their own agreement with Davis.

Seller and purchaser have agreed to a purchase price of $27,650.00, payable as follows:

1. $1,000.00 paid on January 28, 1989
2. $9,000.00 payable on the signing of this agreement, receipt of which is herewith acknowledge by seller
3. $5,000.00 payable on March 1, 1989
4. $12,650.00 in the form of a four-year amortized note attached to this agreement

Seller and purchaser have further agreed that the above purchase price shall be accounted for as follows:

1. $14,000.00 for furniture, fixtures, and equipment
2. $13,000.00 for patient files and information
3. $630.00 for security deposits
4. $20.00 for seller's agreement not to compete

Seller agrees to assist purchaser in becoming familiar with the operation of the practice and in attempting to retain as many of the practice's patients as possible. Seller will undertake this on a "best effort" basis without compensation. For this purpose he will be physically present at the practice for the month of February 1989, during the following hours:

Mondays 1:00 P.M. until 7:00 P.M.
Wednesdays 1:00 P.M. until 5:00 P.M.
Fridays 1:00 P.M. until 3:00 P.M.

Purchaser agrees to hold seller harmless for any claim which may arise out of purchaser's treatment of any patient during this period of "joint work." Seller will remain available for telephone consultation with purchaser regarding any patients seller treated, for an undetermined period of time. Seller will not require compensation for any such consultations, assuming the time required on his part remains reasonable.

As an inducement for purchaser to purchase the practice, and in consideration of the stipulated compensation above, seller agrees not to open another practice within a radius of ten (10) miles from the practice for a period of two (2) years starting with the date of this agreement. Neither seller nor purchaser is aware of the exact distance from the practice to Missouri College or its satellite clinics. This non-compete agreement shall not in any way prohibit seller from accepting any assignments, functions, and/or duties from Missouri College (where he is on the faculty and staff) now or in the future. Should any assignment from Missouri College be, or become, in conflict with this non-compete agreement, purchaser herewith expressly agrees to seller's right to execute such assignment, functions, and/or duties.

Purchaser expressly agrees that the practice, as herewith sold or as it may develop hereafter, shall be collateral against default in their obligations under the attached note, until said note has been paid in full. Seller and purchaser agree that this written agreement constitutes the entire agreement between them. No verbal statements made by seller or his adviser(s) in this transaction shall have any bearing on the execution of this agreement.

Signed, this 31st day of January, at Canada, Missouri.

For Seller: For Purchaser:

_____   _____
Jeffrey Y. Jones, D.C.   Sherri Mayfair, D.C.

                                               _____
                                               Susan Choo, D.C.

Witness to the signing:

_____

At the time of the writing, Drs. Mayfair and Choo have been operating the practice for sixteen months. Business has not always been good for them. Both they and Dr. Jones are happy about the transfer, though. All parties concerned feel that the transition was a good one. Dr. Davis stayed with South Side Clinic for four months after ownership transfer and then moved his practice about ten miles away. The agreement between Dr. Davis and the new owners is shown in Appendix E (Sample Agreement Two).

Because the banks had refused to lend money to Dr. Choo and Dr. Mayfair, Dr. Choo chose to approach her parents for the $10,000 needed to purchase the practice. Her father lent her the money without any kind of repayment agreement. Three months after purchasing the practice, the x-ray machine failed a state inspection. Drs. Choo and Mayfair had already been concerned about the quality of the x-rays and requested an inspection to determine how to improve the operation of the machine. The financial burden of replacing the x-ray and installing an automatic developer at the same time caused Dr. Choo to return to her father for the needed amount of the loan, by now approximately $29,000. The amortization agreed on was a ten-year schedule at 11 percent interest. Besides the $330 the clinic is paying Dr. Jones, it is also paying Mr. Choo $450 each month.

After a tough few months in the middle of 1989, patient count, fees for services, and collections all started to increase slowly. At this writing, the practice is averaging $8,000 in services and collections per month. The practice is and always has been a cash practice. Patients pay for services and file their own insurance claims. Drs. Choo and Mayfair have considered accepting insurance assignment to increase patient count, but feel that the increase in expenses and the delay in payments are not worth the small anticipated increase in revenues. They are satisfied with the current growth trend. Their business plan anticipates payment of decent salaries to them at the end of the third year in practice. Current figures indicate that growth is faster than planned.

The Tax Factor

During the negotiations, tax considerations for both the seller and the purchasers played a role in the final structure of the agreement. Dr. Jones had paid for "goodwill" in his purchase of the practice in 1978. Accountants define goodwill as the difference between the price paid for the practice and the book value of the assets purchased. Therefore, goodwill cannot be depreciated, and the purchasers' adviser strongly suggested against it.* Instead he advised payment for the patient files. These can be amortized, and as a result will assist the new owners with income taxes over the next few years.

A business consists of a number of components. The Internal Revenue Code treats each component separately for tax purposes at the time of sale or purchase. State revenue codes commonly follow federal law. Some of the more common components transferred in the sale of a business are equipment and furnishings, supplies, office leases (premium paid to assure lease), leasehold improvements, real estate, accounts receivable, goodwill, patient files, and restrictive covenant (non-compete). How these components are handled, obviously, is contingent on whether you are the seller or purchaser. Please realize that this list is not intended as advice in specific situations, and that tax law changes frequently. A competent tax adviser should be consulted in each practice purchase or sale situation to maximize your tax benefits.

---

*AUTHORS' NOTE: This was the situation at the time of the case. Today, goodwill can be depreciated.

11

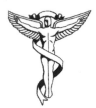 **Running the Office**

The business office is the nerve center of the practice. Patient scheduling, billing, accounts receivable management, insurance submission, practice promotion, supply organization, patient follow-up, public relations, troubleshooting, and last but not least, keeping the practice busy and on schedule are responsibilities this part of the organization handles in a routine day.

Record Keeping

Each section of the business department interacts with the others. The patient's appointment is first entered on the schedule book. After service is received by the patient, the fee for the service goes into the patient accounting program and the amount collected is recorded as well. Accounts receivable amounts will then be billed to the patient and may also go through insurance procedures. A percentage of patients will be considered worker's compensation or personal injury cases. These cases may lead to depositions and/or court testimony. To aid the smooth and uninterrupted flow of paperwork, it is necessary to use a logical filing system, written reports, and patient-flow management.

Schedule Book

While the patient accounting computer program probably has an excellent scheduling module, we find that in most offices the schedule book is the center of the control panel. (See figure 11.1 for an example of a typical page in the schedule book.) A complete understanding of how to schedule patients is needed. To utilize the doctor's time most efficiently, guidelines must be developed:

- Don't spread out appointments. Cluster them when possible, without overlapping. You want to look busy, but at the same time, you do not want to make patients wait very long. A cardinal rule: Their time is just as valuable as yours.

- The sample schedule sheet is set up at five-minute intervals by using all three columns for each time slot. This allows latitude in time allotment per patient. Initially, more time per patient will be available, perhaps ten minutes. But if the practice is to increase, that time period should drop to five minutes. Of course, each patient varies, and the time required may vary according to the patient's changing status. Five-minute intervals allow for additional patient scheduling, for example, while a new patient is being worked up. Don't fall into the trap of taking great periods of time with each patient just because you have the time. As your practice increases, those patients will feel cheated on the time you take. If you are used to taking twenty to thirty minutes per patient, there is no way your practice will grow. It is hard to break an established habit.

- New patients: Allow one hour, and let the patient know how long the visit will take. You can schedule one or two patients for the time while the new patient is filling out forms. You can also schedule one or two patients in during the new-patient workup if you have a CA (Chiropractic Assistant) to assist in the procedure.

- Allow thirty minutes for report of findings (ROF), if utilized.
- Allow one extra time slot if x-rays or exam will be needed.
- Use a coding system for the schedule so that you can tell what is going on at a quick glance. Abbreviate and mark the following in red by the patient's name: RE-E (re-exam), ROF (report of findings), NP (new patient), RE-X (re-x-ray), and N/S (no show). As each patient comes in, mark the schedule with a green dot or a √ mark to show that the patient has arrived. Mark off each time slot needed (scheduled for new patients, re-exams, and so forth.) by drawing a line through it.

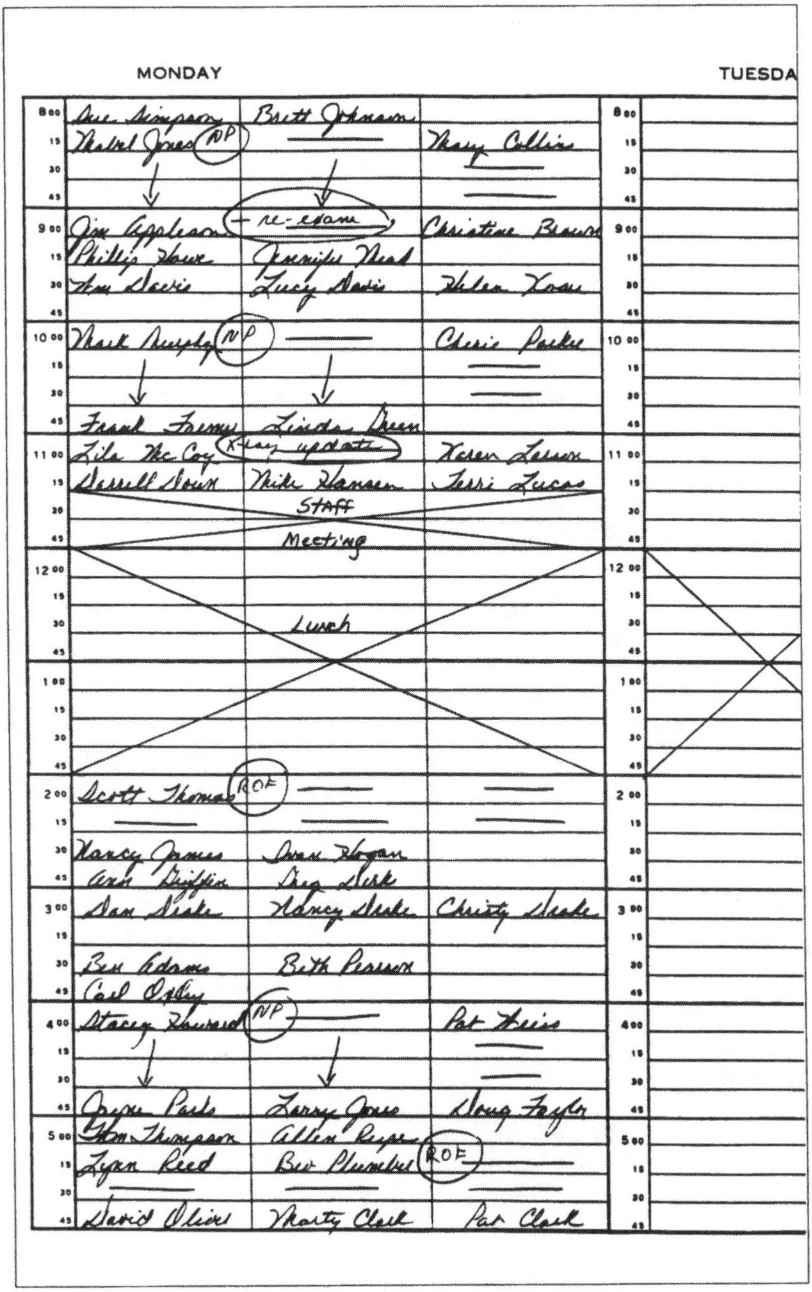

Fig. 11.1. Sample schedule sheet.

- Mark off time for lunch breaks, days off, holidays, and out-of-the-office appointments.
- When a patient does not keep an appointment, mark no show (N/S). Follow up with a call within thirty minutes of the scheduled appointment. If no answer (NA), call later that workday or early the next morning. Be sure to mark N/S and the calls that have been made in the patient's file.
- When a patient drops from care, send out a retrieval or reminder letter.
- If the patient will not be seen in more than one month, use a post-card recall system.
- It may be necessary to call the day before an appointment if the patient forgets easily. (You'll know who they are.)
- Reset practice goals once planned levels have been attained. The importance of working toward goals was discussed in Chapter 1. As an aid, try keeping graphs showing, for example, total patient visits per month, new patients per month, collections month to month, services month to month. The graphs will clearly display progress toward goals and make the central function of management easier.

You can never document too much. If a patient has dropped from care without your recommendation, make a note on the patient's chart. Develop a followup system for contacting patients to determine why they have dropped from care. If there is an account balance, arrange to collect it. If there is still no response, send out a letter of discharge. This formally acknowledges that the patient is discontinuing care and releases you from any responsibility.

Fee Schedule

Post the most frequently occurring charges in the lobby area so the notice is visible to all who enter the office. Include spinal adjustment, after-hours call, exam fee, and any family discount. A complete fee schedule for all services should be posted so that only your office personnel can see it, for easy reference. Since almost all billing is done using Current Procedural Technology (CPT) and International Classification of Diseases (ICD) codes, make sure that the codes are with the appropriate description on the fee schedule. Have the manuals near the checkout desk in case the assistant or you need to refer to it in special procedure situations. Fees to include are:

- Spinal adjustment
- After-hours spinal adjustment
- House call
- Family plan (optional)
- Child fee (optional)
- Therapy
- Cold packs
- X-ray (by size of film)
- Supplements
- Exam: New Patient, Limited, Comprehensive, Athletic
- Blood work
- Reports
- Expert testimony

A fee slip should be attached to each patient's chart or travel card. Commonly, the patient accounting program can print these, individualized with the appropriate patient information; some offices still use the preprinted superbill approach. The services performed are written in or marked with a check mark. The patient returns this travel slip or superbill to the front desk for checkout. This will reduce interruptions by your staff to confirm charges. If a patient receives a service at no charge (N/C) be sure to let him or her know. ("Mrs. Johnson, the ultrasound you had today is normally $10, but since this is your first therapy, there is no charge.") Everyone likes to get something free.

Communicate the office's financial policy to the patient during the first visit, and repeat it as necessary. This policy is in reality a contract between you and the patient. The policy will answer questions such as whether you require full payment on the first visit, whether the patient has insurance or not, or whether you require a 50 percent payment of first day's total. If exceptions to the policy are made, you, the patient, and the appropriate staff members must know what the agreement is. Will a per-visit copayment be made, or will the patient be paying at the end of each week or once a month in case of chronic or preventative care?

Collection

The financial policy will include the collection policy. Set the procedure and follow through with it. Many professionals consider the term "collections" to apply to "problem" accounts. It is much broader. Collections refers to the receipt of payment for services rendered. Ninety percent of patients will pay the doctor without anything but the asking. Five percent of patients intend to pay, but are temporarily incapable of doing so. These patients deserve special arrangements. Three percent of patients intend to pay, but never get around to it. The physician will probably write off or forgive charges for them. Only two percent of patients have no intention of paying for services rendered. The doctor and staff are responsible for spotting this last group as early as possible and, in an appropriate manner, terminating services.

The financial policy and the collection policy should be in writing and communicated to all staff and patients. Requests for exceptions to the policies need to be carefully reviewed and evaluated. Granting of special arrangements needs to be the exception rather than the rule. Collection effort starts with requiring the new patient to fill out the forms completely. While few physicians and staff realize it, much of the information on the new-patient forms is helpful in collecting. Such items as name, address, telephone, spouse, employer, spouse's employer, patient and spouse social security numbers, emergency contacts, are all necessary when the new patient turns out to fall in the "bad bunch" described earlier.

If acceptance of assignment of insurance benefits is part of the financial policy in certain situations, the patient still should be asked, regularly, to pay the standard 30 percent of charges (more on this in Chapter 12). Occasionally, phone calls need to be made to attempt to collect from patients discharged from care. Collection calls are the least favorite office responsibility, but a necessary one when accounts have become delinquent (thirty days or more overdue, showing no payment). The hardest part is initiating the voice contact. The staff member must remember to be courteous, but firm. Be in control, and do not argue. Do not make accusations, always be professional. Two sample phone conversations follow.

The cooperative patient

Office: Hello, Mrs. Johnson, this is Pat from Dr. White's office. I am calling in regard to your account status.

Patient: Yes, I am sorry that I have not sent in a payment.

Office: I would like to assist you in keeping your account current. When can I expect a payment?

Patient: I can send a payment by Friday, May 3.

Office: We would like to keep you current. Can we expect a payment of $——? (Try for a least 50 percent of what patient owes.)

Patient: I can't pay $——, but I can pay $——. (This figures out to 30 percent.)

Office: I can accept that amount, Mrs. Johnson, and I will look for your payment on Friday, May 3. Thank you for your cooperation in this matter.

The uncooperative patient:

Office: Hello, Mr. Jones, this is Pat from Dr. White's office. I am calling in regard to your account status.

Patient: Yes, hello, Pat.

Office: Our office has sent you two statements and we have not heard from you. At this point your account is considered delinquent.

Patient: I have been waiting for my insurance company.

Office: Are you aware, Mr. Jones, that your copayment is expected on a regular basis? You agreed to pay your copayment every two weeks. We haven't received a payment from you in six weeks. In order to return your account to current status, we will need to have your payment of $—— in the office by Friday of this week.

Patient: I do not intend to pay until I have heard from my insurance company.

Office: Mr. Jones, may I remind you that the arrangement of payment is between your insurance company and you? Dr. White agrees to assist you with your insurance provided you maintain your copayments. You are responsible for the services the doctor has provided. This office is more than willing to work with your insurance, as long as your copayment is kept current.

Patient: Have you heard from the insurance company?

Office: No, I will check with them by Friday. If there is a problem, you may need to intercede. I need a payment of $—— on Friday to return your account to current status. When you come in I will have contacted your insurance company. Dr. White has helped you regain your current health status and wants you to maintain it.

Patient: I will be in Friday afternoon.

Office: I will go over your account with you at that time. Thank you for your assistance in this matter.

Keep an activity log to record all the calls made and the actions that are taken on an account, or agreements reached and promises accepted from the patient. This keeps the file in order and avoids small notes that get lost in the patient's file. Be cordial on the telephone, but also be in control and be specific. Set a date when both parties agree to have a payment made (you can encourage postdated checks). Collection letters should be developed and mailed when appropriate. If desired, a working relationship with a trusted collection agency may be developed to use as a last resort.

Patient File System

There are two common approaches to maintaining patient files: the envelope file and the file folder:

Envelop file: This system keeps all patient records in the large file, sometimes called a jacket. This file goes to the adjusting room with the patient each visit. It is labeled with last name first, first name last, middle initial, account number. Full-sheet forms are used. The file is in sections; the chart or clinical file includes all notes taken and the listing of subluxations, recorded on a continuation sheet. This system offers space efficiency for storage. The full-sheet continuation sheet offers more space for notes. It is helpful (although not necessary) to keep separate business and insurance files.

File folder: The file folder system keeps all patient forms in one file, frequently with a number of dividers. Colored-letter labels are used. A travel card, which goes to the adjusting room with the patient, may be used with this system. All the information you will need in the care of your patients can be found on the card: name, address, payment agreement, major complaint, diagnosis, history, x-ray and view(s), x-ray findings, positive orthopedics, subluxation listings, and clinical notes. An initial-care label indicates the year. The travel card offers a more streamlined form to transport with the patient. One drawback is that you must keep a separate file holder to store the travel cards.

Patient records need to be kept for at least seven years, longer in some states and in case of minors.

Patient Care Forms

Many forms for documenting or prescribing care are available commercially at low cost. Always use only those forms which are imprinted with the business name, doctor's name, address, and phone number. Today, many offices design and print their own forms using computer word processing or specialty programs.

Release of Patient Information

Any part of the patient record that leaves the office must be copied and placed in the patient's file. Make sure your staff understands, without question, that all patient records, files, information, and x-rays remain the property of the office or practice. Never, at any time is it permissible to give information from the files or x-rays to anyone, including the patient, without observing the following conditions:

- The patient has signed a release authorizing the office to release x-rays, file, or information. (This can be done in the office in person by the patient or by mail from the organization to receive the file copies.)
- Should there be an account balance, it is good policy to use the occasion to request payment in full.

Patient Procedures

Efficiency and common courtesy are not mutually exclusive. It is possible to create office procedures which provide an efficient operation and a high level of patient care.

Patient Traffic Patterns

Efficient intraoffice traffic flow is crucial to avoid delays, interruptions, and forgotten patients. To make it work, you must rely on everyone's doing his or her part, and, when necessary, stepping in to assist. Remember that the patient always comes first. Before agreeing to rent or lease office space, or before accepting an office building design, is the right time to consider the options. Once the space has been constructed or built out, little can probably be done to improve patient traffic flow.

Patient Protocols

Patient protocols are designed to assure that minimal professional standards of care are met. In addition, because they result in clear, well-delineated actions on the part of the doctor and staff, which the patient observes, they become silent marketing tools. The patient becomes comfortable with the office, the personnel, and the procedures, and will therefore speak highly of the office to others. Some time invested in developing these protocols and standards, in communicating with the staff and the patients, will allow for clear and precise communication for all parties involved. This allows patients to understand that you have expectations of their cooperation in the recuperative process. We know that good health is not just the absence of disease, we need to educate the patients so they come to understand and accept those concepts. It starts the moment the patient walks in the office for the first time. It shows in the consultation, history you take, the examination you perform, the x-ray and lab studies you order, the report of findings and spinal health care classes (extended consultation) you present. Be organized and meticulous, you have been entrusted with caring for another human being.

Some Specific Procedures:

New patient enters office. The patient fills in a history form, is escorted to the doctor's office and introduced; the door is closed. After consultation, the patient may then go on to any one or more of the following: x-ray, exam, and adjustment. If an assistant helps with the exam and x-rays, one or two patients can be seen by the doctor.

Current patient enters office. The chart is pulled and dated. (If two patients arrive simultaneously, the one scheduled first goes first; walk-ins will understand that they must be worked in.) The patient signs in, is escorted to the adjusting room; the doctor is notified. The patient returns after adjustment to the front desk with fee slip, makes payment, and schedules the next appointment. If the assistant is busy with therapy or x-rays, the doctor schedules the patient and receives payment. (If this is a new patient, the assistant should go over the payment policy.)

If there are two assistants in the office, one should be designated to flow to the back to assist the doctor, and the second assistant (usually insurance) designated to cover the front desk. The first assistant should have a professional (medical) or paraprofessional background.

Phone Etiquette

The image you create on the telephone represents the practice. The telephone is the primary public relations source for the practice. Speak directly into the receiver. Write down all messages with date and time; deliver them to the appropriate party. Note if a return call is needed. Determine which type of call the physician prefers to be interrupted for and which will be returned later. Messages should be in writing or relayed by the assistant out of hearing of other patients. Don't argue with patients. Clarify problems and try to reach a mutual agreement. If the assistant is unable to reach an agreement, he or she should arrange for the physician to respond to the patient by some agreed-upon time. Following are some sample telephone calls:

> Patient: I need to speak to the doctor.
> Office: The doctor is with a patient right now. May I take a message and have the doctor return your call?

> Office: Good morning, Dr. White's office, Pat speaking.
> Patient: How much does the doctor charge for office visits?
> Office: Have you been under chiropractic care recently?
> Patient: No.
> Office: Dr. White prefers to schedule a consultation with prospective patients. That way the doctor is able to determine what your needs are. At the time of the consultation the doctor will review the fees.
> Patient: That sounds good.
> Office: When may I schedule your consultation with the doctor?

> Patient: (New patient) I want to schedule an appointment with the doctor.
> Office: I have (give two appointment options) open. You should allow one hour for your first visit. (The visit may not take quite that long, but by allowing an hour, you won't feel rushed.)

Always remember to smile when talking on the phone. Your voice carries your mood and facial expression.

Supplies and Equipment

The state of your equipment is a direct reflection of your skills as a doctor in the patient's eyes. Buy new equipment when possible, you are investing in the life expectancies of the equipment. In the long run, it is better to buy high quality. Make sure that used equipment is in excellent condition. Don't allow the appearance of running the office on a shoestring, even if that is exactly what is happening. The most important priority is keeping your overhead as low as possible, yet low overhead should not equate with low quality. Overhead can make or break the practice. An ideal overhead is 30 percent of gross revenues; if you are running at 60 percent or more, you will be in financial trouble, depressing chances of practice growth and survival.

Be organized in purchasing supplies and equipment. Develop a list of supplies, equipment, furniture, and fixtures you will need. Each room will have its own requirements. The rooms to consider include reception room, doctor's office, the consultation room, business office, adjusting room, dressing room (optional), and restroom.

Several supporting departments will be used in the diagnosis and care of your patients. They are exam, x-ray, physiotherapy, and a laboratory. In addition, a secondary support in the care of your patient will be your orthopedic inventory. Ordering and maintaining these supplies is usually taken for granted until the tool or orthopedic support you need is missing or out of stock.

Once your practice has opened, designate one person for the reordering of supplies. Start an index file showing product, company, address, telephone number, contact person, and the price per quantity.

Develop an inventory file for all supplies, indicating who the supplier is, price and quantity, and any other needed information.

12

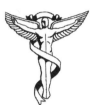 **Getting Paid?**

When the authors talk to students at, or recent graduates from, the various colleges about their experience in the Health Centers, we occasionally hear that they had a superb time at the outreach clinic. They tell us glowingly about the benefits of chiropractic, about how it can assist people with both physical and mental troubles, about the wondrous works they did using neurological concepts, and so forth. We, of course, are delighted to hear this information and observe the commitment such an experience creates in the practitioner. Often, when we notice that the recitation is nearing an end, we ask a rotten question: "What did it teach you about running a practice?" Some return to the clinical concepts. We stop those. Some frown because they notice the direction our interest is taking. Most just stare at us blankly. Would life not be superb for all of us if we could operate a chiropractic office the way we learned at the Harbor Light Clinic?

Reality really does hand out hard knocks. No practice will succeed if it does not charge for services rendered and collect those charges. Many young and inexperienced doctors just do not have the confidence to charge a fair price for the services they render. Others, being poor because of the time they spent as students, have too much sympathy for the patient's presumed financial constraints. If those attitudes were based on reality, it might be understandable, but too frequently that is not the case. The following scenario played out not long after one of the authors started teaching at a chiropractic college.

Robert Ward, a senior student, stopped me in the hallway to introduce his young bride of three years. They were very pleased to announce that since he was now a trimester eight student she could quit her job and prepare herself to assist in running the office. My frown did not stop the rest of the story. Jane (the bride) could afford to quit working because, after five years as an international operator for AT&T (annual income $28,000 plus, in 1984), she had nine months' maternity leave with full pay coming. That would cover the time frame required for Robert to finish school and open the office five blocks down the street. They had signed the office lease (1,000 square feet at $1,400 per month). My frown deepened, was noticed, and they attempted to reassure me that everything would be all right because Jane's dad had guaranteed a $50,000 bank loan. Of course the baby (yes, she really was pregnant) would come to the office with them every day, the architect ($4,500 fee) had designed a crèche in a nice, light corner room. After all, they noted, in the beginning the office won't be so busy that Jane can't take half an hour regularly to breast feed the baby and play with it. No matter what argument or question I presented, I could not induce them to reconsider some of the decisions that had been made. She would quit her job, it was to be a family practice.

Fast forward about ten months. The baby was beautiful and so was the office. Nothing but the best, most expensive equipment and supplies. Baby cried all the time she was in the crèche so she normally was on her mother's arm or lying peacefully on the floor of the business office next to mom. Some time spent with Robert seemed to indicate that things were going well (his statement). In the first month and a half since the office opened they had attracted seven patients, all with low back pain and neurological deficits. Robert would do an excellent exam, take x-rays, try to explain the condition and the recommended care to the new patient, but was puzzled that he could not convince a few of the patients to return for care. The first office visit was priced at an average of $350, return visits at $50 (remember this scenario plays out in 1984, not in 1997). Dr. Ward did feel, though, that something was not quite developing the way he had envisioned it. Could I provide a little advise, please? Before I could respond with some questions and (hopefully) answers, the buzzer sounded and Robert excused himself—that was the signal that the patient was ready to be adjusted. Sitting in his office, looking at the gorgeous mahogany desk, credenza, and bookcase, I tried to figure out how to let him know that he had broken a few cardinal rules of starting a practice. Just as I finished formulating some penetrating questions, Robert returned, rather apologetically, to let me know they were leaving the office for the day. (It was 10:30 A.M. on Tuesday and the only patient scheduled for today was now dressing to leave. "Why hang around the office, we have other things to do and want to get home early today.") Would I please think about the issues and maybe get back to them sometime soon? Consenting, I walked out of the doctor's office, looked around, and noticed that the patient (clearly a successful businessman, if dress is any indicator) was approaching the checkout desk. As he smiled at Jane, he pulled his checkbook and pen out of his pocket. "Jane, how much do I owe you?" he said. The response astounded me: "Oh, John, don't worry about paying now, we'll catch up later." John (of course) smiled and walked out. Hoping to make a difference, I asked Jane why she did not take the check John was ready to write. "Oh, he probably can't afford it, we certainly couldn't." I walked out of the office and found the theme for my lecture on the way to campus: Rudi's first rule of practice management: take cash, check, or credit card. Needless to say, the office closed six months later, Robert and Jane Ward moved (yes, the baby, too) to the state of Washington where they declared bankruptcy five months after arrival. Robert is still a chiropractor today, employed in a high-volume PI practice for the last twelve years. When I talked to him by phone last year, he was bitter—chiropractic never kept its promise to him. By the way, the baby is fine; she is a pretty young lady doing very well in middle school. Jane went to work last year selling and arranging flowers for the local florist.

Financial Policies for the Office

The above true story plays every day all over the country. The sad part of the story is that it does not have to work this way. Smart business management would cause one to make sure that in the beginning the overhead is low, the office small, and the opportunity of a "spousal postgraduate scholarship" be accepted upon being offered. Inexpensive does not equate to low quality. The office can be laid out and furnished without spending tremendously large sums. Clinical competence is a prerequisite for a successful practice; a willingness to do some "fast learning" in the business area is also. In other chapters we develop the concepts of management and overhead control, here let us review the financial policies.

Proper collection policies start with an understanding of the health-care contract between the patient and the doctor. While the contract most often is implicit, it behooves the physician to make it explicit if there is any doubt that the new patient understands it. A good, well-designed and well-presented new patient consultation can clear matters up for many patients. The contract, stated in plain English, says that the doctor will provide the best possible advice and services and the patient will pay the fees charged for those services. Therefore, it is quite acceptable to expect payment at time of services. Cash on delivery is a very common concept in today's economy. If a patient presents good evidence that financial arrangement may be required, it is always possible to make the concession to assist the patient in collecting reimbursement from third-party payors such as insurance companies. The highest possible portion of the fee should be collected at office visit checkout. Family budget plans work well with responsible individuals. Try to spot the person who has no intention of paying the bill as soon as possible in the relationship. There is no law which states that the chiropractor, or any professional for that matter, has to give away services without compensation. There is a law which states that once the health-care contract has been accepted by both parties, certain procedures must be followed to terminate it. Therefore, letters dismissing a patient from care must be carefully drafted.

Probably the first concern of a new practitioner is to establish a fair fee schedule. Using publications such as relative value schedules or *Fee Facts* can help with this. Fair trade practices acts in most states allow for the creation of multiple-level fee schedules as long as the classification of the patient is done on an appropriately distinguishing basis. Discounts for cash payment are allowed under most fair trade practice laws, but may be against insurance regulations in some states. Check with a competent attorney or contact the secretary of state's office to determine the rules of the game. Should a patient build up a balance on account, early and proper intervention is the best policy. In Chapter 11 we provided some telephone conversation scripts which do a fine job of developing cooperation with such patients.

Insurance Company Relations

The submission of insurance claim forms is a service which can be provided for patients. It may be an incentive to the new patient to select the practice for a health-care provider. The keys to an efficient insurance department are the development of direct communication with the patient and the insurance company and an efficient claims processing procedure. Claims can take anywhere from three to ten weeks for processing and payment by the third-party payor. Delays can be caused by incomplete or erroneous information, improper terminology, or the wrong code usage on the claim forms. In fact, insurance companies make it clear that the cause for delay in the largest number of cases is incomplete or missing information on the HCFA-1500. Make sure that the patient understands that insurance is an agreement between the insured (your patient) and his or her insurance company. The patient is totally responsible for any fees for service which have been incurred. Your office will gladly assist by preparing necessary reports and forms to assist in collection. If assignment is accepted, it is the patient's responsibility to pay for deductibles and coinsurance portions, as well as any reimbursement or portion of the fee the insurance company denies. On the initial visit, discuss the office collection policy. Most insurance companies have a copayment, typically 10–30 percent, and a deductible that must be satisfied on a yearly basis. The patient is responsible for these amounts to the practice. The assistant must learn to ask if the patient will pay by check, cash, or credit card. Obtain a point-of-service credit card terminal from the bank and follow the procedures for Visa and MasterCard charges. The bank will charge a small fee for having a terminal and typically 2–4 percent of the charges deposited is incurred as a system service charge. On the first visit, review the charges and explain all office policies. This should be done privately if at all possible. If a financial agreement (or payment schedule) needs to be arranged, record it and have the patient sign it.

A good habit to develop is having the patient sign an "authorization to pay doctor" when sending in insurance claims. Place this authorization in the patient's file, and send a copy with the first claim. Thereafter write "signature on file" on the claim forms submitted for the same occurrence. Claims should be submitted frequently—weekly, twice weekly, or daily, depending on volume of claims handled. Many new practitioners erroneously wait until the claim reaches a minimum amount or covers a number of visits. They believe they are saving postage this way, and hope for a good feeling when the large check finally arrives. Sending small claims clearly does cost more in postage. But, consider this thought: Would you rather receive twenty $35 checks daily, five days a week, or one $3,500 check once a week? Are there benefits to having a smoother cash flow?

Insurance verification is the process of confirming coverage, deductibles, and coinsurance percentages with the insurance company. Some companies will verify coverage only to the insured (the patient). In such cases, it is recommended that a detailed verification questionnaire be given to the patient during the first visit. It must be returned, completed, on the next visit. The staff member receiving it should verify that the patient signed and dated the form. Besides providing information about insurance coverage, this approach has the advantage that the patient cannot deny being aware of the portion of the charges that must be paid out of pocket.

As a rule in assignment of benefit cases, establish the "patient portion" of the services 10–15 percent above the insurance policy's coinsurance. There are a number of reasons for this. First, it improves cash flow. Next, it builds a cushion in the patient's account in case deductibles are applied or charges are reimbursed at a reduced level by the insurance company. Finally, compare the patient's reaction to receiving an overpayment check from the physician with his or her reaction to receiving an unexpected invoice because insurance reimbursement was miscalculated.

Coding for Diagnoses and Services

The authors notice a hesitation on the part some chiropractors to become familiar with the CPT and ICD coding manuals. There is probably a historical reason for this in the profession, but it is high time in the late 1990s to move beyond old prejudices. Every practice should have at least one set of manuals and at least the doctor and the office manager need to be conversant with the philosophy and structure of the systems.

Codes numerically identify the service performed or diagnosis identified for each patient. The Current Procedural Terminology (CPT-4) is used for professional services and the International Classification of Diseases (ICD-9) for diagnoses. Most insurance companies require the use of these codes and will deny claims submitted without their use. It is frustrating if payments are not coming in or are delayed as a result of oversight. Be aware that Medicare and Medicaid require the use of these codes, and that some Health Maintenance Organizations (HMOs) are now requiring their own procedure and diagnosis codes. Some offices still use superbills, most use the walk-out receipt printed by the patient accounting computer program. Either can be used by the patient to submit a claim with the insurance carrier, if that is the arrangement made between the patient and the practice. All required information needs to be present on the forms. These include diagnosis codes (ICD-9-CM), services rendered (CPT-4), date and place of service, and the signature of the provider.

Insurance claims, once submitted, must not be left in the "to be filed" tray. To assure prompt handling and payment by the insurance company, "case management" is required. Ten days after mailing the claim, a phone call to confirm receipt is appropriate. It may sound like this:

Receptionist:	Good afternoon, Dependable Insurance.
CA:	This is Sue Smith at Dr. Mayfair's office. Can you tell me who handles the claims for Mega Corp., please?
Receptionist:	One moment, please.
Benefits Clerk:	This is Joan Henry, may I help you?
Sue:	Joan, this is Sue Smith at Dr. Mayfair's office. Do you handle the claims for Mega Corp.?
Joan:	Yes, may I help you?
Sue:	Last week we submitted some claims to you. I'd like to confirm that you've received them.
Joan:	What are the social security numbers?
Sue:	There are two: 1555151515 and 167895555.
Joan:	The screen shows that both were received yesterday.
Sue:	That's great. Joan, can you tell me if you need anything else before you can process these claims.
Joan:	No, it looks like we have everything.
Sue:	Terrific. Joan, thank you for helping me. I appreciate it. Can you estimate when you will be mailing the checks?

Obviously, this call was successful. Now the claims are filed in the tickler file three days after the promised mailing date. If they are not received that day, Sue picks up the phone again:

Joan:	Good morning, this is Joan Henry. May I help you?
Sue:	Joan, this is Sue Smith from Dr. Mayfair's office.
Joan:	Hi, Sue. How can I help you?
Sue:	Two weeks ago we talked about claims for Mrs. Jones

Joan:

Sue:

and Mr. King. You said the checks would be mailed three days ago and we did not receive them in today's mail. I just wanted to check with you to make sure the post office is providing normal service and that something did not delay them in your office. Would you like the social security numbers again?

Joan:
No Sue, I remember talking with you. I signed the checks last Tuesday, so they were mailed. You should have them soon.

Sue:
Thanks, Joan. Have a nice weekend.

Again, a successful contact and a mission accomplished. Sue and Joan are beginning to establish a relationship. This can be very beneficial to the physician and to Sue sometime in the future.

Expediting payments and reducing requests for unexpected insurance reports are essential to all practices. Develop a submission procedure for insurance claims that provides a brief initial report for new patients and an interim report each time an exam is performed. Maintaining good relations with third party payers includes keeping them informed of the patient's status.

Remember that claims are paid by individuals, not companies. Normal human courtesy and pleasant, positive communications work wonders. Using this approach, many providers are consistently receiving claims payment in less than three weeks. Of course there are always the occasional cases where delays occur, but having the majority of claims paid in three weeks is bound to improve cash flow. It is helpful to keep a card file or database containing all appropriate insurance company information, including names and extensions of the benefit clerks and claims supervisors.

Organization is the primary factor in having a well-run insurance department. All forms submitted must have all the required information filled in, correctly. Develop a process that allows for accurate knowledge of the stage claims are in, as, for example, the date when the claim was mailed, resubmission dates, secondary carriers, paid claims. Document activity of claims on ledger cards. Any additional information needed by the insurance company should be followed up on immediately. Any delay postpones payment by the carrier. If it is known that a report may be needed before payment will be issued by the insurance company, send the report in with the original claim submission. Be organized, know the requirements and "DIRFT" (Do It Right the First Time).

Electric Claims Filing

Insurance claim filing can be accomplished by taking advantage of the changes resulting from the computer age. Medicare is close to requiring providers to submit electronically; currently the anticipated effective date is July 1998. In the past the Health Care Finance Administration (HCFA) has postponed similar requirements a number of times, so at this writing, there is as yet no certainty. In addition, several states have either already mandated all insurance claims be filed electronically or are currently preparing for such a requirement. There are a number of benefits to electronic claims submission:

- It makes it easier to complete the tracking of all services for statistical use
- it reduces data entry error as a result of automatic, electronic screening of each claim
- it makes possible faster claims payment with electronic funds transfer
- it reduces missing information and the resultant delays

Before the claim reaches the insurance company's systems all data entry errors have been eliminated, the claim form is completely and correctly filled out. Transmission from the practice to the carrier is accomplished is under 24 hours.

Some terminology and history may be of assistance in developing comfort with the process:

EDI: electronic data interchange; computer-to-computer transmission of information.

ECS: electronic claims submission

Clearinghouse: a computer-based service company which edits the claims according to carrier requirements, and then, once the claim is correct and complete, transmits it to the insurance company electronically.

Edits: the requirements from each insurance carrier that must be met on each claim.

Transmission: information is conducted via a modem attached to the computer and a phone line that connects to a computer in the clearinghouse.

More terminology referring to computers may be found in Chapter 7.

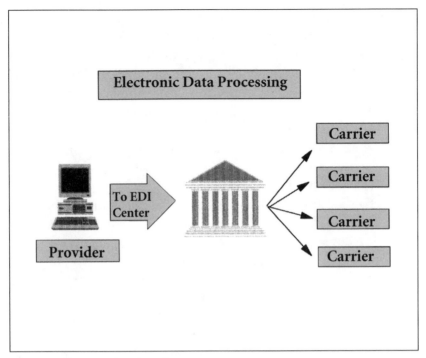

Fig. 12.1. Electronic data interchange.

Electronic filing was started in 1981 by a group of large insurance carriers. NEIC (National Electronic Information Center) was formed and incorporated. The purpose was to develop a paperless system to process claims for insurance carriers and providers. NEIC is the grandfather of clearinghouses. Today dozens of clearinghouses have developed. Understanding the pros and cons for each clearinghouse may be a challenge. The software vendor supplying the program for electronic claims submission will likely have preselected a small number of clearinghouses. If not, their support staff may be able to assist by reviewing each clearinghouse's options and benefits. The schematic diagram in figure 12.1 provides a pictorial representation of the process.

Electronic claims submission provides the following advantages when compared with paper claims submission: reduction of data error, reduction of denied claims and faster turnaround time from the time the claim leaves the office. In order to accomplish this process a computer system and appropriate software are required. The software should allow for one-time-only data entry at the time of the patient visit. With well-designed programs, no further data entry will be required. Because of the ease of this process, we find practices transmit claims daily or at least weekly— definitely an improvement over the paper approach.

Should a practitioner be uncomfortable with the concepts and the process, an option exists in almost all towns: the billing service. These are independent businesses which, for an additional fee, will input the claims into their computer and transmit them through the clearinghouse to the insurance company. Normally, an employee of the billing service stops by the practice once each week to pick up the information necessary to file the claim.

Medicare

Medicare is a federal government benefit program for individuals who have reached the age of 65. Two other groups of individuals are eligible: those who meet specified qualifications of disability or terminal kidney disease. The last two groups represent only a very small portion of the Medicare population. Chiropractors, as physicians, may provide services to Medicare beneficiaries and must then submit a claim for the patient under Medicare, Part B. The Health Care Finance Administration (HCFA), the federal government agency which administers the Medicare program, requires that providers submit the claim for benefits, even if the patient/ beneficiary has paid cash for the services. The program provides reimbursement, to the patient or the provider, for outpatient services, subject to an annual deductible. The reimbursement paid is 80 percent of "approved" charges. For chiropractors, currently the only approved charges are for spinal manipulation. HCFA is considering approving other charges for services by chiropractors at the time of this writing. In order to have manipulations approved, a current x-ray of the area of the spine must be on file in the chiropractor's office. HCFA and its regional payors prefer that all providers agree to become "participating" providers. In our experience, this limits the flexibility of the practice in a number of ways, and therefore, we generally recommend against it, even though the reimbursement level is approximately $1 more per office visit. The disadvantages to the chiropractic office are just too overwhelming, when compared to the advantages, for us to take any other stand at this moment. A "nonparticipating" provider may collect from the patient but must have each patient sign a medically unnecessary statement (MUS form) at each treatment.

Claims must be submitted using form HCFA-1500 with the appropriate ICD-9-CM and CPT-4 codes. Medicare supplement policies, issued by commercial insurance companies and designed to integrate with Medicare, may reimburse services which Medicare doe not pay for.

The authors strongly recommend that the doctor or business manager sit down with each patient and explain the Medicare benefits carefully. Review the appropriate forms with the patient and have those signed if appropriate.

These are our suggested guidelines for each review with the Medicare patient:

- Medicare requires an x-ray to prove "medical necessity" for the manipulation. This is the only way Medicare will pay for adjustments.
- Medicare will pay only for adjustments. It will not pay for x-rays, exam, therapy, supports, supplements, or the like.
- When submitting a claim one of the first three CPT codes for spinal manipulation must be used.
- If the patient does not want an x-ray taken, have him or her sign a waiver (see figure 12.2). This form states that the patient has been notified that Medicare is not expected to pay for the adjustments. The patient is acknowledging having received this information by signing the form.
- When submitting the claim, make sure to report the office fee for the service provided, not just the amount Medicare will approve.
- Have the patient sign an HCFA form for a "signature on file" to be placed in his or her file. Without this, the patient must sign each form.
- Medicare does not recognize the ICD-10 codes; it still requires ICD-9 codes.
- Make a copy of each patient's Medicare card and maintain it in the patient file.
- Medicare ID numbers end with a letter, for example, A, B, D. If the Medicare coverage is not under the patient's number, make sure the file indicates who the Medicare beneficiary is and what the relationship of the patient to the beneficiary is.
- Medicare patients also need to sign a waiver when the services rendered may not be paid by Medicare according to the guidelines given. For example: too many adjustments for diagnosis.

- There no longer is a defined acute status period. All care is determined on an individual basis by "medical necessity."
- The patient should pay for the office visit at time of services, and reimbursement will be mailed by the Medicare payor directly to the patient (this assumes that the chiropractor is a nonparticipating provider).

Medically Unnecessary Service Release Form

Provider Name & Address

LOGAN COLLEGE HEALTH CENTER

PO BOX 1065, 1851 SCHOETTLER ROAD

CHESTERFIELD, MO 63006-1065

Name of Patient

_____

HIC Number

_____

Please Check (√) Appropriate Box:

☐ **Single Date of Service**

☐ **Extended Course of Treatment:**

Specify Date(s) of Service:

_____

To: _____ From: _____

Medicare will only pay for services that it determines to be "resonable and necessary" under section 1862 (a) (1) of the Medicare law. If Medicare determines that a particular service, although it would otherwise be covered, is "not reasonable and necessary" under Medicare program standards, Medicare will deny payment for that service. I believe that, in your case, Medicare is likely to deny payment for

_____ for the following reasons:

(specify particular service)

_____

_____

_____

Beneficiary Agreement:

"I have been notified by my physician that he or she believes that, in my case, Medicare is likely to deny payment for the services identified above, for the reasons stated. If Medicare denies payment, I agree to be personally and fully responsible for payment."

_____   _____

Beneficiary's Signature   **Date**

Fig. 12.2. Medically unnecessary services release form. This form, promulgated by HCFA, must be used in any situation in which the provider suspects that Medicare may not reimburse for the service provided. Check the Medicare regulations and read the Medicare Flash Bulletin *for updates.*

This special Medicare consultation is a greatly appreciated service. Many elderly become confused when trying to understand their coverage. Failure to follow Medicare guidelines accurately means no reimbursement to the patient, who may be living on a rather low income. Senior citizens often rely on the healthcare provider's office to let them know what is expected of them. It is not unusual for the doctor's office to serve as their bookkeeper.

Worker's Compensation

A worker's compensation patient has sustained injuries while on the job. The employer is responsible for the employee's care and payment for that care. The employee must first report the injury to his or her employer; the chiropractor needs to have the employer's authorization to provide care.

At the initial visit, the patient needs to fill out an incident report. Initial billing should be sent out after the first visit. Statements are sent only to the employer or insurance carrier once the authorization for care has been received. At the time of discharge, document the status of the patient and that the patient is released from care. Account for all services on the ledger and submit the final statement immediately.

Personal Injury

A personal injury case involves a patient who has sustained injury by another person or on someone else's property. The greatest percentage of personal injury cases are automobile related and are referred to the chiropractor by the patient's lawyer in the tort case.

On the initial visit have the patient fill out a case history, incident report, and the insurance carrier information. It is especially important to have an "authorization to pay doctor" signed. Send an initial statement after the first day of care. In personal injury cases partial payment may be received. Many times full payment is not made until settlement of the case, although we advise doctors against entering this kind of relationships with lawyers. The patient should be encouraged to make payments on the account to keep the account current and avoid interest charges. Submission of claims with the health insurance and/or med pay carrier is legal in some states and should then be done. Statements need to be sent on a regular basis to the patient, insurance carrier, and attorney involved. The attorney involved should be willing to execute a signed attorney's lien, guaranteeing payment for services. Be aware, however, that in some states the attorney's lien is a valueless piece of paper—it cannot be enforced. Other states take a more supportive attitude and will force the attorney to back up the financial guarantee the lien represents. Narratives are frequently required in personal injury cases. Reply as soon as possible, but only when requested. Do not volunteer narratives. At the time of discharge, document patient status and release from care. Document all services and send a statement with the discharge note to the insurance company. If a suit is in process, remain in contact with the patient and the attorney to stay aware of the status of the suit.

Depositions and Court Testimony

Occasionally, a chiropractor will be asked to provide expert testimony in a lawsuit. Special attention must be paid when scheduling and billing for depositions and court testimonies. Lost time and revenue, and office stress, are often caused by poor communication with the attorney requesting assistance. Some chiropractors enjoy this work and develop a procedure to follow with every legal case. By developing a regular procedure for working with attorneys on depositions and court appearances, problems will be minimized and communication of all sorts clearly executed. Problems which do develop are often due to a lack of communication between offices. Clear communication with the attorney about the established office procedures, fee schedules, and guidelines, in advance of accepting an assignment, assures easy cooperation between professionals and proper compensation for time and effort invested. Cancellations often occur within hours before a scheduled meeting; it appears to be the nature of working with attorneys. Should this occur, it causes an empty schedule book, without offsetting billable time for the deposition or testimony. Billing for such unproductive time, if so agreed to in the acceptance of the assignment, avoids this loss of revenue, and frequently avoids last-minute cancellations in the first place. For any deposition or testimony, it is crucial to appear on time and to be well prepared. It may take a few sessions before the physician becomes comfortable with the atmosphere, the thought processes, and the demeanor of those involved in lawsuits. The antagonistic environment is not for everyone. The best advise we can provide is to try it a few times. If it remains uncomfortable, decline future opportunities.

Managed Care Organizations

Much has been written about managed care organizations and their growth as a market force in the health-care industry. Still, we find much misconception about them in the chiropractic profession. The following information may be helpful to a better understanding. It needs to be clearly understood that if a health-care provider accepts a managed care contract, the health-care contract with the patients described above is replaced by a three-party agreement: the patient, provider, and payor are all part of the same contract. This is a new situation, which imposes certain restrictions on the provider, and the patient.

The oldest form of a managed care organization is the HMO. The first ones started in the late 1920s and were a minor market force until the passing of the federal HMO Act of 1974. This law mandated that employers provide HMO memberships to those employees who so request, if the employer provides group health insurance as an employee benefit. In addition, to assure that there were an adequate number of HMOs, the law provided financial support for startups by the federal government. In the middle 1970s, the HMOs had become somewhat of a factor in the health "insurance" market, and solicited a reaction from the traditional insurance companies. This reaction came in the form of Preferred Provider Organizations (PPO), which grew quickly in number and market penetration due to marketing structure and sales force of the insurance companies. A PPO attracts physicians to its network by offering to list them in the policies (marketing factor) and to promise the insured (the patient) that their only cost will be a small, per visit charge. The provider agrees with the PPO to accept a reduced reimbursement to allow the insurance company to state that care is assured at the small co-pay amount. In the early 1980s these two organizations had generated enough market power that the physicians who did not belong to either organization started noticing an effect on their practices. Some of those doctors reacted by creating their own form of managed care organization, the Independent Practice Association (IPA). Due to the low marketing and business savvy of the doctors, many IPAs went bankrupt and were absorbed into HMOs or PPOs. Some HMOs also fared badly from a business and financial point of view and were bought by insurance companies. Thus was created the now common form of managed care organization, the Point of Service network (POS). This approach is a combination of one or more of the above organizations with commercial insurance to provide choice to the patient at the time that health-care services are needed. The patient can see one of the preferred providers, or go to the HMO clinic, or visit the doctor of choice. Reimbursement for the care provided depends on the choice of service made. In addition, the POS, because of the availability of the traditional insurance benefits, started the trend to providing out-of-area coverage now commonly seen in all forms of managed care.

Managed care organizations typically reimburse providers in one of three ways: fee for service, case-based reimbursement, or capitation. There are still some HMOs in the country that employ the doctors and compensate them on a salary basis. Historically that was the HMO approach. In the chiropractic profession, we most commonly see the fee for service (reimbursement based on the doctor's fee schedule) and the case reimbursement approach (based on the diagnosis; a case has a stated value which the doctor receives through the combination of the office visit copayment and the payment from the managed care firm). Rarely do we see capitation in the chiropractic profession, or, for that matter, in the other small group and solo practitioner health care fields.

Managed care has experienced tremendous growth in the 1980s and 1990s. A review of some statistics indicates the change: in the St. Louis metropolitan area less then 20 percent of the population was covered by managed care in 1990, this grew to 40 percent in 1993, and the best available estimates are 65 percent in 1996. That is not the whole story though. The states of California, Oregon, and Arizona have almost 95 percent of the population covered in managed care. Today almost all managed care organizations have similar characteristics. They have an office visit copayment, have utilization review, and they have pre- or concurrent authorization of care.

To become (and remain) a provider in a managed care organization, the doctor needs to submit to a credentialing process. Providers (that is, you) are reviewed for performance (clinical judgment and results), quality (most often based on patient and peer satisfaction with service and care), and value (economic/financial results). The overall judgment of the managed care organization is based on the Value Matrix; the MCO wants "Best Practices" providers. The value matrix is based on two axes: cost of care and quality of care. The best practices providers provide high-quality care at low cost. While most providers resent this cost versus quality push, we find it interesting to note that in managing their own practice they should take exactly the same point of view. Each doctor wants to provide patients with the best possible care at the lowest possible cost to the practice. Somehow, when others force us to keep that commitment, we are displeased. To put it in the terms of one managed care organization (American Chiropractic Network, Inc.):

> Clinically we want the chiropractor who has skill in gathering information, demonstrates effectiveness in using diagnostic methods, has competence in diagnosis, exhibits good judgment and skill in implementing treatment and competence in providing continuing care, is effective in patient-physician relationships and accepts responsibilities of a physician.

To review the concept of credentialing, the following questions and answers are helpful:

- *What is it?* An assessment and validation of the qualifications of the providers.
- *Why is it?* Quality assurance from the plan's point of view: Quality providers give quality care and service at economic value. In addition, quality meets the guidelines and requirements of the customer (employer) and guarantor (U.S. government).
- *How often does it take place?* Annually or biannually?

The credentialing process consists of several parts: a licensing check (verified with state); confirmation of graduation from chiropractic college, confirmation of malpractice insurance and a report of claims against the provider, obtaining evaluations of the provider from government benefit programs (Medicare and Medicaid) and other insurance companies, a curriculum vitae showing a minimum of three to five years of provider work history, and, finally, a site visit. Once the provider is contracted, the evaluation continues. Records are maintained to indicate the cost (reimbursement and number of visits per case) and quality (most often determined by patient and peer satisfaction) of care provided. Thus, in recredentialing, in addition to the above steps, a performance review is included.

Managed care is here to stay. We do not necessarily advocate that all chiropractors, or other health-care providers for that matter, should contract with an MCO. We do advocate that before condemning something, an understanding of the phenomenon be developed. Whether managed care is a satisfactory approach for all concerned—the patient, the provider, and the real payor (employer or tax payor)—is yet to be determined. What is clear is that the health-care inflation rate is declining from the astronomical figures (20–40 percent per year) of the mid- and late 1980s. Many observers credit managed care with this accomplishment. Many observers also indicate that the pendulum of cost cutting may be swinging too far the other way. Experience teaches us that natural cycles will cause a happy medium to be found. Once that situation has developed, all of us can again return to the work, attitudes and ethics we prefer: let's do the best job possible for the patient the first time.

In the previous few pages we have discussed the ways the doctor can expect to be paid for services rendered to the patient. While we have spent most time and attention on the third-party pay structures that exist, we feel compelled to point out this was by environmental force. We strongly believe that the best possible world for all concerned is for the chiropractor to operate a "cash" practice. It is a little harder to "sell" to some patients, but in the long run the patients who "buy" the concept are more committed to their health, and better understand the value of the services provided. The trouble that exists with this approach is in the mind of the practitioner. We have visited with large numbers of very successful practitioners who are generating very substantial incomes with this approach. A pleasant side benefit may be that a large insurance office staff, and the attached cost, is not required. Remember Rudi's first rule of practice management: Patient, how do you expect to pay for my services—cash, check, or credit card?

Part Four

The Hard Stuff: Getting the Money to Start

13

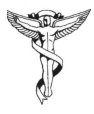 # Accounting for Small Business

The first time most nonfinancial professionals listen to a conversation between accountants, bankers, investment counselors and the like, they are convinced that, without spending a nickel on travel, they have landed in some foreign country. Jargon exists in all professions, but those guys can really use English words with different meanings! In this chapter their language will be introduced.

The first part of this chapter will look a lot like a foreign-language vocabulary list from the campus bookstore. Precision of terminology is not the purpose; understanding concepts is. The list is not alphabetized, as that would only add to the confusion. The next part discusses the construction of financial statements. The last part introduces the concepts and techniques of cash-flow projections and risk analysis. Our purpose is not to make the reader into an accountant, instead we only wish to provide the minimum level of understanding that appears to be a prerequisite for communication with accountants. Before proceeding it is appropriate to take a look at the purpose of accounting.

Purpose of Accounting

One wonders at the use of accounting. Is it worth the effort to understand accounting? What does accounting do to help us? There are three basic purposes for accounting:

- Internal use: Accounting generates reports to management (for the control function in PPBIC) on a timely basis. These reports are of a consistent form and in a unified measure (dollars).
- Friendly outsiders: Other (nonactive) owners and creditors (trade and financial) will sometimes require information on the progress and creditworthiness of the business. (Ask yourself the question: Would you lend me money if you had no idea whether my corporation is capable of paying back the principal you are lending, and the interest you expect to earn on the money lent?)
- Government: The Internal Revenue Code states that a business shall keep those books that allow it to provide the information required on tax returns. In addition to the Internal Revenue Service, a number of other governmental organizations may have similar requirements. For example, state and local governments may require that certain information be available for inspection in order to determine that state income taxes, state property taxes, local property taxes, merchants' and manufacturers' taxes, sales taxes, and the like, have been paid appropriately.

Definitions

The purpose of this part of the chapter is to provide some basic knowledge. It is structured in an informal style in the expectation that this approach will aid understanding.

Financial statements: A group of four papers in standardized accounting format providing information on the current financial status of a business. The four statements are the balance sheet, the income statement, the funds statement, and the reconciliation of retained earnings.

Balance sheet: The part of the financial statements of a business that, as the name indicates, must balance. Perhaps you have seen one of those old-time apothecary scales known as balances—the same principal applies here. The balance statement describes the current financial status (of a business or person) and is valid only for the moment it is created (more on this later).

Asset: That which the business owns. Always shows up on the left side (let's really confuse you—sometimes on the top) of a balance sheet.

Liability: That which the business owes. Always shows up on the top right side (or the middle) of the balance sheet.

Owner's equity: The difference between assets and liabilities. Always shows up on the bottom right side (or the plain bottom) of the balance sheet. The term "owner's equity" (also called net worth) applies to a proprietorship; it is changed to "partnership capital" or "stockholder's capital" or "equity" in the other business forms. There is such a thing as negative owner's equity.

The Accounting Equation: If the above three items made sense to you, this one is easy: Assets = Liabilities + Equity. The result of these few terms can be seen on page 152 of this chapter.

Liquid asset: At least we know what an asset is, but liquid? And on paper? Money (greenbacks) is liquid. It can be exchanged easily for other items. Therefore, any asset that can be turned into money (read: sold) quickly is called liquid. Because interpretations of "quickly" may differ, ninety days has been established as the norm. Thus, because I can sell my inventory of vitamins in a three-month period (even if I have to take a loss), inventory is a liquid asset.

Fixed assets: Those assets that will always be part of the business; they are a necessity to run the business. It is possible that the individual item changes over time, but an item like it will always be present. For example: a treatment table will always be part of a chiropractic office. Maybe it is a flat table in the first few years, to be replaced by a more expensive hi-lo table when the business has generated enough cash to afford it, but there will always be a treatment table. In the long run, of course, all assets can eventually be liquefied (sold), but the time frame (ninety days) is the dividing line here.

Miscellaneous assets: Those things owned that fit neither of the above asset descriptions. They are not intended to always be part of the business, nor can they be turned into cash within ninety days. A typical example for a chiropractic office is the rent security deposit paid at signing of the office lease. Some accountants prefer the term "other assets" for this category.

Short-term liability: Liabilities can be divided in a similar manner to assets. The point of separation in liabilities is one year, however. In other words, if you expect to pay off a liability within one year, it is considered to be short term.

Long-term liability: Those liabilities which are to be, presumably by preagreement, paid off some time after one year from the date of this balance sheet.

Stockholder's equity: If you have the annual report of your favorite corporation handy, you will note that there are quite a few entries or accounts (we'll define both shortly) there. You are likely to see:

    Common stockholders' capital: The amount paid for common stock by all the owners at original issue at

    Par: The price of the stock stated on the stock certificate.

    Preferred stockholder's capital: Preferred because dividends are payable to these people before dividends can be paid to the common holders.

    Dividend: The stockholder's portion of the corporate profit.

    Retained earnings: The profits from previous years' operations that were not paid out by the company but kept inside for investment.

    Paid-in capital: Something that shows up if, at original issue, a stock with a par value sells for more than that stated amount.

We are really speaking accounting now! We know the terminology of the balance sheet. Let us venture on:

Income statement (formally P+L/Profit and Loss statement): The part of the financial statements of a business that, as the name indicates, calculates the income of the business. Profit or loss is reflected on the bottom line (hence the expression, "the bottom line").

Revenues: The top portion of the income statement reflecting all moneys taken in by the business as a result of operating the business (so, not loans or capital additions).

Expenses: A section of the income statement showing the amounts spent on accounts (to be defined shortly) necessary for the generation of revenues for the business. Typically, this includes all expenses which the Internal Revenue Code says are deductible from revenues in the calculation of taxable income.

Cost of goods sold: Just as the name implies, the cost to the business of those goods (for physicians we are talking about vitamins, nutrition supplements, braces, pillows, and so forth) that are sold by the business. A distinction here is made in cost to the patient and cost to the business. Cost of goods sold reflects the cost of the material to the business, not the selling price by the business to the patient.

Depreciation: A method of reducing the value of a capital asset over a period of time. This can be done on a unit basis (as an example, if an x-ray instrument is said to be good for 24,000 "clicks," and if it costs $12,000, then each picture represents a reduction in value of the instrument by fifty cents), or on a time-of-service basis (a hi-lo table is expected to serve the practice for five years; it is acquired at a cost of $5,000, and as a result each year reduces in value by $1,000). These two examples are of straight line depreciation. Tax law allows for accelerated depreciation, but we will leave the calculation to the accountants.

Amortization: The same concept as depreciation, but is applied to intangible assets (for example, value of patient files purchased).

A basic knowledge of arithmetic, you'll notice, comes in handy, not only in speaking accounting, but also in the running of the business. If fingers and toes turn out to be inadequate, adding machines, calculators and/or computers will be of assistance. Most people would be so confident of the foreign language of accounting by now that they might try to display their knowledge in appropriate social settings. There is a danger to this: at each social setting there is likely to be a frustrated accountant present. That person will not allow you to outshine him or her, so some more basic terms need to be defined:

Account: Originally a piece of paper, typically in the form of a T-account (see below), on which all transactions of the business were recorded. There is an account for each individual person or organization that the business has transactions with (such as patients), as well a for any of the assets, liabilities, equities, revenues, or expenses.

T-account: An old-fashioned term used to indicate that all business accounts were kept on balance-type pieces of paper with left and right sides, and that at all times, but especially at the end of an accounting period, the account should balance. The balance sheet is a form of a T-account.

Ledger: A book, or grouping of sheets, of accounts; also the individual sheet in such a book, as in "each patient has an individual ledger."

Debit: A term which for some reason creates tremendous confusion in speakers. It means simply the left side of the T-account.

Credit: The opposite of debit and as a result, the right side of any T-account.

Accounting period: All accounting is done for a given period of time; a 12-month period for proprietorships and partnerships (tax law requires it to be a calendar year). All financial statements reflect the business situation at the end of one year, and, as a result, at the beginning of the next accounting year. Financial statements are sometimes drawn up more frequently than annually. The accounting period can be subdivided into quarters, the quarters into months.

Entry: A name for anything entered in any spot on any accounting piece of paper.

Pro forma: Means "using the form of." As an example, a pro forma balance sheet is frequently created when starting a business, even though few assets, liabilities, and equity entries will be reflected. It is used to predict what the planned results of operations will look like after the stated period.

We are really almost done. There are many more terms, some of them used in everyday American English, which we shall not attempt to define or describe here; therefore, only a few more.

Funds: All things of value, including money, flowing through the business, no matter what the source. Be careful using this one; "money" and "funds" are not interchangeable. Feel free to ask the person using the term "funds" for a definition.

IRS: Internal Revenue Service, an agency of the United States government charged with the collection of all internal taxes. These initials create a sense of uneasiness in many a law-abiding taxpayer. Yet, because the IRS is a U.S. agency, it does not have the notorious subjectivity of its equivalents in other countries. It works according to published rules and regulations and under U.S. court supervision. A taxpayer and the IRS may disagree, but that does not give the IRS the power to break the law.

IRC: The Internal Revenue Code of 1954, as amended (over and over and over again); the law which is the basis for, among other items, federal income taxes.

Journal: A book of original entry, meaning that in this book all transactions which occur in a firm are recorded for the first time. At a later time, and possibly by a different individual, each transaction is then transferred to (read: rewritten into) the ledger accounts.

Double-entry (typically followed by "bookkeeping"): A method of making original entries in the books that not only creates the journal entry, but at the same time allocates the appropriate amounts to the correct ledger accounts.

One (w)rite: A special form of double-entry bookkeeping, using a pegboard and carbon-paper approach, which creates the journal entry, the ledger card entry, and the invoice or receipt. Probably the trade name of a manufacturer originally, now rather generically used.

Disbursement: What, you don't carry a burse anymore? Oh, well, a burse is a coin or currency wallet. Now does the word make sense?

Cash flow: Yes, exactly as you thought. For more (and more, and more, and more) about this matter you will have to read the last part of this chapter.

Receivables: Simply enough, those funds yet to be received but already legally earned by the business. The name of the liquid asset account that in many professional offices is the most active account.

Payables: The opposite of receivables, meaning those funds the business currently holds but already owes to another. The name of a short-term liability account.

South Side Clinic • Jeffrey Y. Jones, DC.
108 Main Road • Anywood, Missouri 63199

Acct #	Account Name	Acct. Type	Level	Type	General
1	**Assets**	Asset	1	General	
11	*Current Assets*	Asset	2	General	1
111	Petty Cash	Asset	3	Detail	11
112	Checking Account	Asset	3	Detail	11
113	Savings Account	Asset	3	General	11
1131	MO Bank CD	Asset	4	Detail	113
1132	Money Market Account	Asset	4	Detail	113
114	Patient Receivables	Asset	3	Detail	11
115	Inventory	Asset	3	Detail	11
12	*Fixed Assets*	Asset	2	General	1
121	Furniture & Fixtures	Asset	3	Detail	12
122	Clinic Equipment	Asset	3	Detail	12
123	Leasehold Improvements	Asset	3	Detail	12
131	Depreciated Furniture & Fixtures	Asset	3	Detail	12
132	Depreciated Clinic Equipment	Asset	3	Detail	12
133	Amortized Leasehold Improv.	Asset	3	Detail	12
15	*Miscellaneous Assets*	Asset	2	General	1
151	Security Deposits	Asset	3	Detail	15
152	Patient Files Purchased	Asset	3	Detail	15
2	**Liabilities**	Liability	1	General	
21	*Current Liabilities*	Liability	2	General	2
212	Accrued Expenses	Liability	3	Detail	21
214	Bank Credit Line	Liability	3	Detail	21
215	Accrued Taxes	Liability	3	General	21
2151	Accrued Payroll Tax	Liability	4	Detail	215
2152	Sales Taxes Collected	Liability	4	General	215
21521	Sales Taxes Received	Liability	5	Detail	2152
21529	Sales Tax Pd. on Purch.	Liability	5	Detail	2152
2153	Social Security Tax Withheld	Liability	4	Detail	215
2154	Medicare Tax Withheld	Liability	4	Detail	215
2155	Income Tax Withheld	Liability	4	Detail	215
2156	State Inc. Tax Withheld	Liability	4	Detail	215
2157	City Inc. Tax Withheld	Liability	4	General	215
22	*Long-Term Liability*	Liability	2	General	2
221	Bank Notes	Liability	3	General	22
2211	Missouri Bank	Liability	4	Detail	221
3	**Net Worth**	Capital	1	General	
31	*Owner's Net worth*	Capital	2	General	3
311	Dr. Jones' Net Worth	Capital	3	Detail	31
32	*Owner's Withdrawals*	Capital	2	General	3
321	Dr. Jones' Withdrawals	Capital	3	Detail	32
33	*Current Period Profit*	Capital	2	Detail	3
4	**Revenues**	Revenue	1	General	
41	*Patient Revenues*	Revenue	2	General	4
411	Manipulation Office Visits	Revenue	3	Detail	41
412	PT Fees	Revenue	3	Detail	41
413	Lab Fees	Revenue	3	Detail	41
414	X-ray Fees	Revenue	3	Detail	41
415	Sales Orthopedics and Nutritionals	Revenue	3	Detail	41
416	Patients Receivable Adjustment	Revenue	3	Detail	41
417	Exam Fees	Revenue	3	Detail	41

Fig. 13.1. Chart of accounts (continued next page).

418	Report of Findings	Revenue	3	Detail	41
419	Other Office Charges	Revenue	3	Detail	41
42	Cost of Services	Revenue	2	General	4
423	Lab Expenses	Revenue	3	Detail	442
424	X-ray Expenses	Revenue	3	Detail	42
425	COGS Orthopedics/Nutritionals	Revenue	3	Detail	42
49	Miscellaneous Income	Revenue	2	General	4
491	Miscellaneous Revenue	Revenue	3	Detail	49
192	Interest Earned	Revenue	3	Detail	49
493	Finance Charges	Revenue	3	Detail	49
494	Purchase Discounts	Revenue	3	Detail	49
499	Gain/Loss Sales Fixed Assets	Revenue	3	Detail	49
5	**Expenses**	Expense	1	General	
51	*Employee Expenses*	Expense	2	General	5
5110	Salaries	Expense	3	Detail	51
5111	Professional Substitute Compen.	Expense	3	Detail	51
5112	Casual Labor	Expense	3	Detail	51
5113	Payroll Taxes	Expense	3	Detail	51
5114	Group Life Insurance	Expense	3	Detail	51
5115	Group Health Insurance	Expense	3	General	51
	Owner's Health & Accident	Expense	4	Detail	5115
51152	Employee Health & Accident	Expense	4	Detail	5115
5116	Education Expenses	Expense	3	Detail	51
52	*Office Expenses*	Expense	2	General	5
5210	Rent	Expense	3	Detail	52
5215	Utilities	Expense	3	Detail	52
5220	Telephone	Expense	3	Detail	52
5225	Office Supplies	Expense	3	Detail	52
5227	Clinic Supplies	Expense	3	Detail	52
5230	Postage	Expense	3	Detail	52
5235	Dues & Subscriptions	Expense	3	Detail	52
5240	Repair	Expense	3	Detail	52
5245	Insurance Expense	Expense	3	General	52
52451	Malpractice Insurance	Expense	4	Detail	5245
52452	General Insurance	Expense	4	Detail	5245
5250	Uniforms & Laundry	Expense	3	Detail	52
53	*Patient Acquisition Expense*	Expense	2	General	5
531	Patient Educational Materials	Expense	3	Detail	53
532	Newsletter	Expense	3	Detail	53
533	Advertising	Expense	3	Detail	53
534	Clinic Promotion	Expense	3	Detail	53
54	*Financial Expenses*	Expense	2	General	5
541	Interest Paid	Expense	3	Detail	54
542	Bank Charges	Expense	3	Detail	54
543	Depreciation & Amortization Exp.	Expense	3	Detail	54
545	Legal & Accounting Expense	Expense	3	Detail	54
546	Taxes & Licenses	Expense	3	Detail	54
547	Contributions	Expense	3	Detail	54
548	Deductible Car Expenses	Expense	3	Detail	54
549	Credit Card Expenses	Expense	3	Detail	54
55	*Miscellaneous Expenses*	Expense	2	General	5
551	Business Meals & Entertainment	Expense	3	Detail	55
552	Convention Expenses	Expense	3	Detail	55
553	Travel Expenses	Expense	3	Detail	55
554	Patient Refund Expenses	Expense	3	Detail	55
559	Miscellaneous Expenses	Expense	3	Detail	55

Fig. 13.1. Chart of accounts (continued).

Fiscal year: An accounting period. Does not have to run coincident to a calendar year and is typically named for the calendar month in which the fiscal year starts. Proprietorships have always been required to have a calendar fiscal year, and recently partnerships came under the same requirements.

Short year: A one-time possibility. When a corporation first starts business, it is allowed to choose its first fiscal year to be shorter than 12 months.

Personal services corporation: A new term introduced in the 1986 Tax Act. It means that the corporation earns most of its revenues from the personal services of its owners-employees. Probably all health-care providers who incorporate will fall under this definition. Income taxes paid by the corporation are much higher than for nonpersonal services corporations. Uncle Sam is trying to tell us: If you are keeping profit in your corporation (which people might do to avoid or reduce taxes) it will cost you.

Chart of accounts: That list the accountant gave you has a purpose. All accounts are listed with their names and probably each with a number. The accountant uses the numbers because the paper is too small for those account names. Besides, computers are happier with numbers than with names.

Well, it was hard work, but we have successfully completed an introduction to accounting. The best advice is to learn the above list by memorization. This language eventually becomes part of everyday life for the entrepreneur.

Finally, let us review a typical chart of accounts. The one on pages 150 and 151 is for a practice called South Side Clinic. It shows clearly the division into assets, liabilities, and so forth. It shows the short-term and long-term divisions as well as some others. The word "detail" indicates to the accountant that the account is used for journal entries. The "general" accounts do not receive any entries; they receive their values from the underlying detail accounts, sort of like a summarized account. This chart is designed for a chiropractic office, and other health-care providers might receive one with slightly different revenue account names.

The Financial Statements

The chart of accounts leads logically into a discussion of the financial statements. It clearly indicates to the initiated individual the format that the accountant intends to use for the balance sheet and income statement.

When accountants use the term "financial statements," they think about four separate forms: the balance sheet, the income statement, the funds statement, and the reconciliation of retained earnings. The funds statement shows where the monies came from and how they were used. The accounting profession requires that the funds statement be presented in a precise format, one not always helpful to the small business owner. Like the balance sheet, a funds statement always balances, because it is impossible to have received money and not be able to show where it is (this is speaking accountingese, of course; in real life everyone who handles a checkbook or cash drawer knows better).

The reconciliation of retained earnings is prepared for corporations only. Partnerships receive a similar statement, the capital accounts statement. Some accountants will prepare an owner's equity or net worth reconciliation, if specifically asked to. The reconciliation of retained earnings starts with the account balance from the previous balance sheet, adds this year's net income (profit), subtracts any dividends paid out, and ends with the new retained earning account balance (that is, if everything is in good shape). These statements can at certain times provide information helpful to the entrepreneur. Most of the time, however, they are prepared for the tax return and for the accountant's satisfaction.

In the small business, cash-flow management is more important than profit. In the beginning of a practice, when there are few patients and it seems as if the mail carrier brings only bills, cash flow is negative. This period of time is referred to, by the authors, as the Valley of Death. If the business does not have the capital to survive that period and come out on the other side, then business death is a certainty. Therefore, the accountant familiar with the operations of small businesses almost always presents the income statement on a cash rather then accrual basis. Attention to this statement is the most crucial management function in the beginning.

The financial statements reproduced on pages 154 through 157 will assist in understanding what information the balance sheet and income statement can provide. It is important to keep in mind that a balance sheet, by definition, gives only a monetary picture of a continuous flow of activity. One can compare it with taking photographs of a rapidly flowing river. No matter how quickly the photographer can snap the shutter, any two successive pictures will show differences. The same is true for a bal-

Balance Sheet

Jeffrey Y. Jones, DC　·　108 Main Road　·　Anywood, Missouri 63199

December 31, 1996

Description	This Period	%	Year to Date	%
Assets				
Current Assets				
Petty Cash	$0.00	0%	$100.00	0%
Checking Account	$7,662.26	51%	$32,753.24	14%
Savings Account	$0.00	0%	$0.00	0%
Patient Receivables	$7,414.08	49%	$200,179.20	86%
Inventory	$0.00	0%	$78.85	0%
Total Current Assets	$15,076.34	100%	$233,111.29	100%
Fixed Assets				
Furniture & Fixtures	$0.00	0%	$14,805.81	6%
Clinic Equipment	$0.00	0%	$55,249.48	24%
Leasehold Improvements	$0.00	0%	$0.00	0%
Total at Cost	$0.00	0%	$70,055.29	30%
Less Depreciation				
Depreciated Furniture & Fixtures	$0.00	0%	($14,805.81)	(6%)
Depreciated Clinic Equipment	$0.00	0%	($55,249.48)	(24%)
Amoritized L/H	$0.00	0%	$0.00	0%
Total Depreciation & Amoritization	$0.00	0%	($70,055.29)	(30%)
Total Fixed Assets	$0.00	0%	$0.00	0%
Other Assets				
Security Deposits	$0.00	0%	$500.11	0%
Patient Files Purchased	$0.00	0%	$0.00	0%
Total Other Assets	$0.00	0%	$500.11	0%
Total Assets	$15,076.34	100%	$233,611.40	100%
Liabilities				
Description	This Period	%	Year to Date	%
Current Liabilities				
Accrued Expenses	$0.00	0%	$0.00	0%
Bank Credit Line	$0.00	0%	$0.00	0%
Accrued Payroll Tax	$0.00	0%	$0.00	0%
Sales Taxes Collected	$0.00	0%	$8.54	0%
FICA Withheld	($4.24)	(0%)	$35.95	0%
Income Tax Withheld	($13.00)	(0%)	$104.00	0%
State Income Tax Withheld	$10.00	0%	$37.00	0%
Total Current Liabilities	($7.24)	(0%)	$185.49	0%
Long-Term Debt				
Missouri Bank	$0.00	0%	$0.00	0%
Total Long-Term Debt	$0.00	0%	$0.00	0%
Total Liabilities	($7.24)	(0%)	$185.49	0%
Net Worth				
Dr. Jones' Net Worth	$0.00	0%	$197,406.34	85%
Dr Jones' Withdrawals	($2,822.07)	(19%)	($155,900.88)	(67%)
Current Period Profit	$17,905.65	119%	$191,920.45	82%
Toal Net Worth	$15,083.58	100%	$233,425.91	100%
Total Liabilities & Net Worth	$15,076.34	100%	$233,611.40	100%

Fig. 13.2. Balance sheet (continued next page).

Last Year	%	Variance	%
$100.00	0%	$0.00	0%
$32,370.01	16%	$383.23	1%
$0.00	0%	$0.00	
$164,851.82	83%	$35,327.38	21%
$78.85	0%	$0.00	0%
$197,400.68	100%	$35,710.61	18%
$14,805.81	7%	$0.00	0%
$55,249.48	28%	$0.00	0%
$0.00	0%	$0.00	
$70,055.29	35%	$0.00	0%
($14,805.81)	(7%)	$0.00	0%
($55,249.48)	(28%)	$0.00	0%
$0.00	0%	$0.00	
($70,055.29)	(35%)	$0.00	0%
$0.00	0%	$0.00	
$500.11	0%	$0.00	0%
$0.00	0%	$0.00	
$500.11	0%	$0.00	0%
$197,900.79	100%	$35,710.61	18%

Last Year	%	Variance	%
$0.00	0%	$0.00	
$0.00	0%	$0.00	
$0.00	0%	$0.00	
$202.96	0%	($194.42)	(96%)
$103.49	0%	($67.54)	(65%)
$44.00	0%	$60.00	136%
$144.00	0%	($107.00)	(74%)
$494.45	0%	($308.96)	(62%)
$0.00	0%	$0.00	
$0.00	0%	$0.00	
$494.45	0%	($308.96)	(62%)
$246,405.02	125%	($48,998.68)	(20%)
($202,446.66)	(102%)	$46,545.78	(23%)
$153,447.98	78%	$38,474.47	25%
$197,406.34	100%	$36,019.57	18%
$197,900.79	100%	$35,710.61	18%

Fig. 13.2. Balance sheet (continued).

Income Statement

Jeffery Y. Jones, DC • 108 Main Road • Anywood, Missouri 63199

For the period January 1 through December 31, 1996

	This period	%	Year to Date	%
Office One Services				
Mainpulation Office Visits	$4,328.32	17%	$44,627.93	17%
PT Fees	$7,440.00	29%	$71,734.00	27%
Lab Fees	($54.50)	(0%)	$22.50	0%
X-ray Fees	$1,000.00	4%	$12,750.00	5%
Exam Fees	$760.00	3%	$7,008.15	3%
Report of Findings	$0.00	0%	$0.00	0%
Other Office Visits	$220.60	1%	$3,122.60	1%
Sales Ortho/Nutr	$0.00	0%	$37.76	0%
Office One Total	$13,694.42	54%	$139,302.94	52%
Office Two Services				
Manipulation Office Visits	$3,801.87	15%	$47,988.51	18%
PT Fees	$7,460.00	29%	$82,860.00	31%
Lab Fees	$0.00	0%	$0.00	0%
X-ray Fees	$1,300.00	5%	$18,460	7%
Exam Fees	$1,210.00	5%	$11,410.00	4%
Report of Findings	$0.00	0%	$0.00	0%
Other Office Visits	$125.00	0%	$2,709.60	1%
Sales Ortho/Nutr	$0.00	0%	$37.76	0%
Office Two Total	$13,896.87	54%	$163,465.87	61%
Revenues				
Combined Fees	$27,591.29	108%	$302,768.81	114%
Patients Receivables Adjustments	($2,018.31)	(8%)	($36,190.76)	(14%)
Total Revenues	$25,572.98	100%	$266,578.05	100%
Miscellaneous Incomes				
Interest Earned	$29.28	0%	$512.88	0%
Miscellaneous Revenue	$0.00	0%	$1,521.39	1%
Rent Received	$0.00	0%	$0.00	0%
Gain/Loss Sales FA	$0.00	0%	$0.00	0%
Total Miscellaneous Incomes	$29.28	0%	$2,034.27	1%
Cost of Revenues				
Lab Expenses	$0.00	0%	($47.50)	0%
X-ray Expenses	$0.00	0%	$0.00	0%
COGS Ortho/Nutr	$0.00	0%	($822.95)	0%
Total Costs	$0.00	0%	($822.95)	0%
Gross Margin	$25,602.26	100%	$267,789.37	100%

Fig. 13.3. Income statement (continued next three pages).

Last Year	%		Variance	%
$42,215.44	18%		$2,412.49	6%
$65,890.00	28%		$5,844.00	9%
$148.00	0%		($125.50)	(85%)
$11,070	5%		$1,680.00	15%
$6,940.00	3%		$68.15	1%
$0.00	0%		$0.00	
$7,890.55	3%		($4,767.95)	(60%)
$1,614.26	1%		($1,576.50)	(98%)
$135,768.25	58%		$3,534.69	3%
$43,703.10	19%		$4,285.41	10%
$79,680.00	34%		$3,180.00	4%
$0.00	0%		$0.00	
$14,480.00	6%		$3,980.00	27%
$13,560.00	6%		($2,150.00)	(16%)
$0.00	0%		$0.00	
$715.00	0%		$1,994.60	279%
$1,516.77	1%		($1,479.01)	(98%)
$153,654.87	66%		$9,811.00	6%
$289,423.12	124%		$13,345.69	5%
($56,313.28)	(24%)		$20,122.52	(36%)
$233,109.84	100%		$33,468.21	14%
$506.11	0%		$6.77	1%
$10.70	0%		$1,510.69	NM
$16,030.00	7%		($16,030.00)	(100%)
$0.00	0%		$0.00	
$16,546.81	7%		($14,512.54)	(88%)
($84.50)	(0)%		$37.00	(44%)
$275.25	0%		($275.25)	(100%)
($1,226.81)	(1)%		$451.36	(37%)
($1,036.06)	0%		$213.11	(21%)
$248,620.59	107%		$19,168.78	770%

Fig. 13.3. Income statement (continued).

Income Statement

Jeffery Y. Jones, DC · 108 Main Road · Anywood, Missouri 63199

For the period January 1 through December 31, 1996

	This Period	%	Year to Date	%
Operating Expenses				
Salaries	$783.75	3%	$6,817.50	3%
Professional Substitute Compensation	$0.00	0%	$0.00	0%
Casual Labor	$160.00	1%	$160.00	0%
Payroll Taxes	$64.20	0%	$980.71	0%
Group Life Insurance	$0.00	0%	$0.00	0%
Group Health Insurance	$0.00	0%	($10.00)	(0%)
Education Expenses	$0.00	0%	$0.00	0%
Qualified Plan Administration	$0.00	0%	$0.00	0%
Ee Qual Plan Contribution	$0.00	0%	$0.00	0%
Rent	$2,573.00	10%	$30,734.20	12%
Utilities	$162.39	1%	$973.91	0%
Telephone	$329.32	1%	$3,936.20	1%
Office Supplies	$121.60	0%	$1,269.13	0%
Clinic Supplies	$142.73	1%	$1,528.45	1%
Postage	$98.98	0%	$691.57	0%
Dues & Subscription	$0.00	0%	$146.54	0%
Service & Maintenance Contribution	$0.00	0%	$390.53	0%
Repair & Maintenance	$1,161.95	5%	$1,229.95	0%
Malpratice Insurance	$0.00	0%	$1,782.00	1%
Uniforms & Laundry	$0.00	0%	$50.00	0%
Patient Education Materials	$0.00	0%	$20.00	0%
Newsletter	$0.00	0%	$0.00	0%
Advertising	$567.25	2%	$8,931.35	3%
Clinic Promotion	$25.00	0%	$142.00	0%
Interest Paid	$0.00	0%	$0.00	0%
Bank Charges	$23.88	0%	$296.68	0%
Deductible Car Expenses	$0.00	0%	$0.00	0%
Credit Card Expenses	$0.00	0%	$0.00	0%
Depreciation & Amoritization Expenses	$0.00	0%	$0.00	0%
Legal & Accounting Expenses	$150.00	1%	$2,143.50	1%
Taxes & Licences	$650.60	3%	$655.88	0%
Contributions	$0.00	0%	$110.00	0%
Business Meals & Entertainment	$85.76	0%	$516.76	0%
Convention Expenses	$0.00	0%	$99.00	0%
Travel Expense	$0.00	0%	$0.00	0%
Patient Refund Expense	$183.00	1%	$10,732.88	4%
Miscellaneous Expenses	$0.00	0%	$0.00	0%
Total Expenses	$7,696.61	30%	$75,868.92	28%
Net Income	$17,905.65	70%	$191,920.45	72%

Fig. 13.3. Income statement (continued).

Last Year	%	Variance	%
$13,394.75	6%	($6,577.25)	(49%)
$1,093.35	0%	($1,093.35)	(100%)
$148.50	0%	$11.50	8%
$1,210.09	1%	($229.38)	(19%)
$0.00	0%	$0.00	0%
$551.99	0%	($561.99)	(102%)
$0.00	0%	$0.00	0%
$0.00	0%	$0.00	0%
$0.00	0%	$0.00	0%
$30,666.75	13%	$67.45	0%
$1,127.67	0%	($153.76)	(14%)
$5,465.33	2%	($1,529.13)	(28%)
$1,393.13	1%	($124.00)	(9%)
$1,542.45	1%	($14.00)	(1%)
$771.61	0%	($80.04)	(10%)
$149.00	0%	($2.46)	(2%)
$471.78	0%	($81.25)	(17%)
$58.00	0%	$1,171.95	2021%
$1,402.21	1%	$379.79	27%
$0.00	0%	$50.00	N/M
$0.00	0%	$20.00	N/M
$0.00	0%	$0.00	0%
$11,484.50	5%	($2,553.15)	(22%)
$2,610.06	1%	($2,467.66)	(95%)
$0.00	0%	$0.00	0%
$404.99	0%	($108.31)	(27%)
$0.00	0%	$0.00	0%
$0.00	0%	$0.00	0%
$4,469.20	2%	($4,469.20)	(100%)
$2,150.00	1%	($6.50)	(0%)
$569.58	0%	$86.30	15%
$54.00	0%	$56.00	104%
$930.92	0%	($414.16)	(44%)
$300.00	0%	($201.00)	(67%)
$2,366.62	1%	($2,366.62)	(100%)
$8,460.27	4%	$2,272.61	27%
$11.40	0%	($11.40)	(100%)
$95,172.61	41%	($19,303.69)	(20%)
$153,447.98	66%	$38,472.47	25%

Fig. 13.3. Income statement (continued).

ance sheet. Accountants tell us that the function of an income statement is to explain the differences between the two balance sheets. Frequently the explanation becomes so complex that the entrepreneur has no choice but to believe it.

A detailed look at the asset side of the balance sheet shows clearly the separation of assets into current, fixed, and miscellaneous, as was discussed in the previous section of this chapter. By agreement among accountants, all assets are placed on the balance sheet at the lower of cost or market value. Once on the balance sheet, an asset (with rare exceptions) is not revalued. For instance, Dr. Jones bought an x-ray machine when he started the practice and had it installed. The total cost to have a usable x-ray was $18,000. Today, 9 years later, the machine is still listed in the ledger at $18,000 and is part of the clinic equipment value on the balance sheet. It is also clear, however, that some recognition of the reduction in value occurs because of the depreciation. The balance sheet shows the total depreciation on all equipment since each piece was acquired. To see what depreciation is being claimed in the current year, one needs to look at the income statement under expenses.

The liability and net worth side of the balance sheet again clearly shows the expected division of liabilities. Some accountants may be more precise than others and will split the bank loan (or other debt) into two portions reflecting the parts which will be paid this year and those that will be paid later.

The net worth section indicates that Dr. Jones operates a proprietorship by the names of the accounts listed. The equity reflects monies Dr. Jones has invested in his practice over the years.

Withdrawals is a temporary account reflecting what Dr. Jones has taken out of the practice during 1996. The current period profit is also a temporary account showing how much the practice has earned so far this year. At the end of the year (December 31) the accountant will move the balance to the net worth account, so that the new year can be started with zero balances. That is the process indicated when the accountant refers to temporary accounts.

While interesting information can be obtained from a balance sheet, the real value of the piece of paper comes from comparing each account's value with the same account's value prior balance sheets. That comparison will show trends, and thus provide usable management information.

Other valuable information is developed by comparing current account values to the budgeted (read: planned) values. In the experience of the authors, however, few small business owners will prepare a budgeted balance sheet for each year (in fact trying to develop planned or budgeted expenses is hard enough for most of us). Some accountants will calculate a number of balance-sheet ratios. For example, they might present the current ratio. It is calculated by dividing total current assets by total short-term liabilities. It will clearly show whether the business can pay its bills in the next few months. There are a large number of balance-sheet ratios that can be calculated, but the value of them in a small, closely held business is questionable. A cash-flow statement would probably be more helpful than the information provided by all balance-sheet ratios combined.

The income statement revenues section shows clearly what each type of procedure has generated in fees for the doctor. Some accountants will not take the time to keep these in separate ledgers, and will show only an account named "Fees." Obviously this latter approach does not help the physician make financial decisions as easily. The cost of revenues section is what accountants call a section of counter accounts. They reflect the monies spent on lab fees, x-ray solutions, and film, and orthopedic supports that were purchased by the practice to provide services to patients. Some accountants will include these under the expenses section.

The listing of expenses is self-explanatory; all are cash expenses, except for depreciation. Depreciation is what accountants refer to as a noncash expense. Of course, when the asset was bought, money was spent that could not be deducted immediately.

The miscellaneous income section reflects possible ordinary income that is not really a direct result of operating the practice. For example, if Dr. Jones were to sell one of his treatment tables to Dr. New for $2,000, and if the table had been completely depreciated on the practice books, then the account gain or loss on the sale of fixed assets would show the $2,000. It appears that Dr. Jones had an independent contractor for some period of the prior year. We conclude this because of the slightly more then $16,000 in rents received shown in the last year column.

By separating the accounts in sections the owner is presented with a clear picture of what the practice is producing in income, and what portion of the profit (or loss) is generated by other transactions.

Cash Flow

In an earlier section of this chapter, reference was made to the importance of cash flow in the beginning of a business enterprise. We recommend that detailed cash-flow projections be prepared as part of the business plan. A well-thought-out cash-flow projection is a tool that will be of valuable assistance in assuring survival through the Valley of Death.

The importance of cash flow cannot be overstated. It has been said that in starting their practices doctors can make all the business mistakes in the world, as long as new patients keep coming through the front door. This statement points out that in a physician's office cash flow starts with new patients. Let's analyze the statement. New business owners make mistakes. Mistakes in business cost money. Money in a physician's office is collected from patients and third-party payors for professional services rendered. Services can be rendered to patients only. If new patients do not come into a practice with no existing patients, then no services can be rendered, no fees collected, and no mistakes paid for. New patients show up in physician's offices as a result of marketing efforts. The business plan therefore starts with a detailed marketing plan. In this chapter the existence of a marketing plan has been assumed.

The big question, of course, is, who prepares the cash-flow projections? Does the physician need to be personally capable of running these calculations? While the authors strongly recommend a positive response, the answer clearly may be, no. Today's computers and spreadsheet programs are easy enough to operate and to become comfortable with. A few hours invested in learning to operate, and move around in, a spreadsheet program will pay handsome returns during the life of a practice. One of the major values of the cash-flow projection exercise is that it forces the tying together process on the entrepreneur. Until this moment, the future business owner has thought in a compartmentalized manner. Dr. New has made decisions on marketing, on fee schedules, on treatment plans, on renting space, and on buying or leasing equipment, and so forth. Only when the cash-flow projection process is started are all these decisions integrated into one effort.

The cash-flow projection starts with patient revenue projections. For those, the new-patient count for each week must be projected, a new-patient office procedure and average fee need to be decided on, patient treatment programs and returning patient office fee must be laid out, and financial policies must be established. If the intent is to operate a cash practice, it seems reasonable to expect that 50–70 percent of fees will be paid at time of service; if it is to be an insurance practice, 30 percent may be a more appropriate assumption. In either case, assumptions need to be made about the total collection ratio (collections divided by fees for services), and the average delay involved in collection the remainder of the fees. These are just some of the integrating thought processes that are involved in cash-flow projections. Appendix F provides a sample cash-flow projection for a fictitious practice to be started. The authors recommend that each practitioner spend some time analyzing the four pages and developing a similar tool for each endeavor to be started. As can be noted from the business plans and loan proposals in Appendices G and H, the first year cash-flow projection is just the start of the total projections most lenders want to see.

No matter who actually prepares the projections, the starting entrepreneur needs to be able to understand the pieces of paper presented by the office manager or accountant or business adviser. It is immaterial whether cash flow and/or risk analysis calculations are done by hand or on computer (although the computer allows much faster recalculation and updating than manual cash-flow statements, and we question whether anyone really uses paper spreadsheets anymore).

Risk Analysis

Risk analysis is really a "what if" game. It uses changes in the assumptions of the cash-flow projections. Risk analysis is where using a computer for cash-flow projections really pays off. Assume for a moment that the originally planned office space falls through. Now the entrepreneur is considering two possible alternative office locations, but the rent will be $1,000 at one and $750 at the other. The lower-rent space, however, will require approximately $11,000 in improvements before it is usable for the physician. The entrepreneur will have to borrow the additional $11,000, thus increasing the required monthly loan payments. Simply plugging these new figures into the overhead and loan payment columns of the spreadsheet will show the new cash-flow situation instantaneously. This "playing" with the figures is some of the best preparation time the entrepreneur can spend.

Risk analysis, once learned, becomes one of the most useful tools to the entrepreneur in the running of a business. Any time a money decision has to be made, the response can be: Let's check the spreadsheet. Risk analysis is helpful in deciding the timing and structure of equipment to be purchased and real estate to be acquired (the clinic building), as well as in evaluating changes or proposed changes in tax law. It is a systematic, quantifiable way of answering the question, Is a particular risk acceptable?

As a final thought, the authors like to point out that a major result of the time and energy invested in the effort to created a cash-flow projection is the Valley of Death graph which is easily created from the spreadsheet. The answers to a few questions now become clear: How deep is the valley? When will I reach the bottom? When will I reach the other rim? All can be clearly seen on the graph.

14

 # The Silent Partner: Taxation

No business in the United States can be operated without consideration for the silent partners always present. The taxing authorities in this country are many and varied. Every activity, business as well as personal, is subject to some form of taxation at some time. Today, it is not uncommon to hear entrepreneurs complain about being taxed too much. Even though many other countries have higher tax rates, few if any can match the United States in sheer number of taxes and taxing authorities. A listing of some of the more common taxes (Fig.14.1) will make the point more clearly.

Although the list may appear to be complete, be assured that it is not. Even this partial list, though, illustrates that taxes are an important part of everyday business life. As a result, taxes must be dealt with in the PPB as well as the I and C portions of management functions.

This chapter will pay attention primarily to the most common federal taxes, as taxes vary widely among states and localities. Familiarity with nonfederal tax requirements is therefore left to the entrepreneur.

Each business owner should obtain a copy of the *Federal Employer's Tax Guide* (Circular E), as well as its counterpart for the appropriate state. The local IRS office can provide a copy of the federal publication: the state department of revenue can supply its papers. Government entities,

Federal Taxes
    Income taxes
    Estate taxes
    Social security taxes
    Medicare taxes
    Unemployment taxes
    Excise taxes (typically hidden in the price of products)
    Import duties

State Taxes
    Income taxes
    Sales taxes
    Property taxes
    Merchant and manufacturer taxes
    User fees
    Unemployment taxes

Local Taxes
    Income taxes
    Sales taxes
    Property taxes
    Merchant and manufacturer taxes
    Occupancy taxes
    Inventory taxes
    Utility taxes
    Entertainment taxes

Fig.14.1. A partial list of common taxes.

federal, state, and local, offer many publications providing tax information for small businesses, all at no cost. The smart entrepreneur makes certain to stay up-to-date on the topic of taxes.

The authors strongly suggest that each chiropractor owning a practice, or planning on opening one in the near future, obtain a copy of the free IRS publication entitled *Tax Guide for Small Business*. In addition, we suggest that every few years the regularly scheduled IRS seminar for small business owners be attended. Taxes have a major impact on business decisions (although no decision can be made solely on the basis of the tax impact) and business owners therefore need to understand and stay up-to-date on current tax laws.

The subject of federal income taxes always seems to steal the spotlight from other types of taxes. Congress and the president have made no fewer than eight major overhauls of the Internal Revenue Code since 1981. The media have rightfully given the subject of federal income taxes a lot of ink. Newspapers and magazines regularly print articles about proposed changes in the tax laws. They will not provide the detailed information needed in the management of a business, but will, however, indicate when further information and study are required. A look at how taxes come about is helpful in explaining where news organizations find the information for their stories.

The House of Representatives of the United States Congress has the constitutional duty to propose taxes it deems appropriate. The House Ways and Means Committee is where the process starts. The committee writes and then reports out a tax bill, which the House as a whole votes on. Assuming passage in the House, the Senate then takes its turn. It refers the House bill to its appropriate committee, which reports back to the entire Senate with a recommended action. Frequently the Senate makes changes in the House version of the bill. This leads to a joint House-Senate conference meeting. Both houses must pass the agreed-upon document before the bill is sent to the president for his signature or veto. When signed, a bill becomes a law.

The current Internal Revenue Code was enacted in 1954 and has since been amended numerous times. Another revision is being discussed on Capitol Hill and on the campaign trail by the president and the various congressional representatives and senators. It is impossible for an accountant, attorney, or business owner to attempt to predict the result of certain tax change discussions occurring in Washington. Crystal balls are notoriously cloudy and cracked, and therefore, incorrect.

Many entrepreneurs would like the government to notify them of changes in tax law. This, however, is not the government's responsibility. The government publishes the law in the Federal Register. It is the duty of each citizen to know the law, and the Federal Register is available for subscription. The fact that as reading material it is better than a sleeping pill does not relieve the citizen and entrepreneur from his or her civic obligation to know the law. It may, however, be a reason to hire competent advisers in the accounting and legal professions.

Before we proceed, it needs to be stated that this chapter is intended only to provide an overview of some of the tax laws which have an impact on the business owner. It is not intended to serve as a substitute for qualified professional tax advice. This chapter is a summary and does not account for all the rules in the Internal Revenue Code and Regulations. As stated above, only cursory attention can be paid to state and local taxes and tax rules. The taxes we are most concerned with here can be categorized by "what gets taxed" in these groupings: employment taxes, property taxes, sales taxes, and income taxes

Employment Taxes

Employment taxes are those taxes levied on employers as a result of employing people. They are FICA (Federal Insurance Contribution Act), and FUTA (Federal Unemployment Tax Act), and the latter's state counterpart, SUTA.

FICA

The purpose of FICA is to pay for social security and medicare benefits. The tax is levied on wages, salaries, proprietorship and partnership profits, and other kinds of earned income. Any employee, including the stockholder employee, must pay social security taxes of 6.2 percent of wages up to a wage base of $62,700 (1996) and medicare taxes of 1.45 percent on all income without an upper limit. The wage base for social security tax increases annually with inflation, the tax rates (percentages) are adjusted by tax law changes only.

The employer must match the employee's "contributions," doubling the total tax rates to 12.4 percent and 2.9 percent respectively. In other words, the corporation owner-employee with a salary of $62,700 is subject to a total FICA tax of $9,593.10, while any income in excess of this amount is still subject to the 2.9 percent medicare tax. Half of these taxes are paid out of the employee's pocket, half out of the corporation he or she owns.

A sole proprietor and partner must pay the "doubled" tax rates in the form of self-employment tax on the profits of the proprietorship or distributed share of partnership profit. On the personal income tax return, the proprietor may take half this amount as a business expense, or half of the amount may be used as an adjustment to income on the front of the tax return. If the proprietorship employs anyone else, the employee pays half and the employer matches it. Of course, all of the matched FICA tax is a necessary business expense, and thus may be deducted on Schedule C as a tax paid.

FUTA and SUTA (Federal and State Unemployment Taxes)
The purpose of these taxes is to pay federal and state benefits to the unemployed. These are levied on employee wages up to a wage base. These taxes are levied on employers and may not be passed on to employees. In general, the federal government taxes the wage base of each employee up to $7,000 at a rate of .008 or .8 percent, for a maximum tax per employee of $56 per year.

State taxes are generally higher, but rates vary greatly. Most states start a new employer at a rate based on the industry average and then develop a rate for that specific employer over time. If the employer has no unemployment claims filed against the account, the state gradually reduces the rate of tax. Many employers with stable work force eventually achieve a tax rate of 0 percent and thus pay no state unemployment tax.

As stated before, rules vary from state to state, and the state unemployment agency should be contacted to determine whose wages and profits are subject to unemployment taxes. This same organization will provide the tax rate and wage base. In many states, sole proprietors and their family members are exempt. Workers employed as "independent contractors" are sometimes considered employees under state law for unemployment tax purposes.

Reporting and Paying Employment Taxes

Occasionally one hears about a business being closed down because taxes were not paid. Most of the time, it turns out, the taxes in question are unemployment taxes. It seems that the government feels that employers should act as collection agents. The taxes are supposed to be withheld from employee paychecks and matched when required. Therefore, if the employment taxes are not reported and paid as prescribed by law, the tax authorities are neither understanding nor lenient. Many entrepreneurs find this reason enough to hire professional help.

Listed below are some of the most frequently used employment tax reporting forms. The frequency with which they must be filed varies with the amount of money due. It is obvious that the more owed, the sooner it has to be paid.

Form 941 is used to report federal income tax withholding, as well as employee and matching employer social security and medicare taxes. The form is filed quarterly, but deposits may have to be made more frequently. Normally, deposits are made at the bank on a monthly basis. This is required if, at the end of any month, more than $500 in taxes is due, or if the employer has been notified by the IRS. While this amount seems large ($500), almost any chiropractic office with a full-time employee falls under the rule on monthly depositing. Employers with payrolls that are very large should check with an accountant. They may owe deposits more often than monthly. The deposit, a check payable to the bank, must be accompanied by a coupon, Form 8109-B.

The quarterly return (Form 941) and the coupon must both display the employer's EIN (Employer Identification Number). The EIN for an employer is not unlike the social security number for an individual. It is applied for on Form SS-4 from the IRS. Quite simple to complete, the form can be obtained from, and must be filed with, the IRS service center for the location of the employer. Circular E shows all IRS service centers in the United States. Many service centers will accept telephone applications for the EIN and issue one to the business owner during the phone conversation.

The FUTA tax is reported on Form 940 and filed at the end of the calendar year. Taxes may have to be paid on a quarterly basis. The procedure to make deposits for FUTA is the same as described above, a different block checked on the coupon being the only distinction.

Each state has its own array of forms to complement the federal forms for unemployment, income tax withholding, and the like. And, of course, the states add a few extras, like corporate franchise tax reports and sales tax reports. In many cases, county or city government also tax income and require the appropriate returns.

Employees must be notified of their total earnings, withholding, and social security taxes for the year on Form W-2. It must be provided to every employee by January 31 of the succeeding year. Copies are sent by the employer to the Social Security Administration and the state department of revenue.

Independent contractors, those individuals not subject to withholding and social security, receive a Form 1099. There are a number of different versions of this form, each with a different purpose. All report income not subject to withholding. The contractor receives the original and the IRS a copy from the "employer."

Property Taxes

Most state and local governments tax real estate, automobiles, equipment, and other forms of tangible personal and business assets. Some even levy a tax on inventories. Reporting property, filing returns, and paying the tax must be done annually in most states, more frequently in some. Some states and localities require quarterly payment and annual reporting. The department of revenue, business tax bureau, and the county or city government revenue department will be delighted to provide the required information.

Sales Taxes

In many states and localities sales taxes are levied on the type of retail sales made by chiropractors. Nutritional supplements or vitamins, orthopedic support, and the like, rarely are exempt from sales tax. Some states will lower the rate levied on these products when compared to the "ordinary" sales tax rate. Sales taxes are an "agency" tax just like the payroll taxes. Therefore, it is incumbent upon the practitioner to assure the timely filing and payment of sales tax reports and collections.

Individual Income Taxes

To report to Uncle Sam, add up your earned and unearned income and allow certain expenditures or "deductions" (standard or itemized) and a "personal exemption" for each family member, to arrive at "taxable income." The taxable income figure is entered on the tax table to determine the amount of tax. If taxable income is over $100,000, the tax tables are not used, and a tax rate schedule is used instead. This is a quick but accurate description of the Form 1040 process. The only other important factors are credits against tax. A credit is applied directly to the amount of tax owed and is received for specific situations. Child care credit is an example most Americans are familiar with. Federal income tax rates are "progressive," meaning the percentage tax rate goes up as taxable income goes up. Many taxpayers therefore pay attention to the marginal tax rate.

Marginal Tax Rate

The marginal tax rate is the percentage in taxes to be paid on the last $1.00 of taxable income earned in the year. To determine the marginal tax rate, determine "taxable income," enter it on the tax rate schedule, and find the percentage listed opposite the taxable income. For tax and financial planning the marginal tax rate is critical. In 1986, the congressional representatives who sponsored the new tax law made a big deal out of how, by eliminating numerous tax deductions, they could reduce tax rates, but it should be emphasized that tax rates are still high enough that a middle-class business owner must actively pursue tax planning. For 1997 the rate on, say, $50,000 of taxable income, is 28 percent. However, this statement is misleading. The new tax law actually phases out the tax benefits of exemptions and deductions for high-income individuals, creating an actual top marginal tax rate of 39.6 percent.

To illustrate the value of knowing the marginal tax rate, let's consider the case of Dr. Jeffrey Y. Jones and his practice, as presented in Chapter 13. He is a married taxpayer with $46,500 in taxable income from the college and his wife's employment. If, in addition, he operates his proprietorship in 1997, each $1,000 he earned in profit from it would have been subject to tax as follows:

Social security on last $1,000 (15.3%)	$153.00
Federal income tax on last $1,000 (28%)	$280.00
State income tax on last $1,000 (6.0%)	$ 60.00
Total taxes	$493.00

He would have paid 49.3 percent of his profit in taxes. His decision to sell the practice and spend time with his family now not only makes sense from a personal point of view, but from a financial standpoint as well. Dr. Jones's income of $46,500 does not in today's economy put him on easy street. One factor to be remembered is that his income was not near the social security wage base. At $62,700 the 15.3 percent would change to the 2.9 percent Medicare tax in the calculation. If his income were to grow to $147,700 or more, the income tax marginal rate would increase to 36 percent from the current 28 percent, while his FICA tax rate would drop from 15.3 percent to 2.9 percent. State income tax would remain at the 6 percent rate, thus his total marginal rate would drop to 44.9 percent. Not good, but better than his current situation. The moral of the story is that tax planning is important for most business owners. It frequently represents time and professional fees well spent.

An often-asked question is, What must be counted as income? According to the Internal Revenue Service, there are several types of income. "Ordinary" income is fully taxed. One hundred percent of this type of income must be included in the income on the tax return. Some examples are:

- Fees, salaries, wages, bonuses
- Profits from proprietorships and partnerships
- Interest (taxable) and dividends on stock
- Pension payments
- Fifty percent of social security benefits
- Taxable fringe benefits
- Profits on sale of property, stock, bonds, etc.

"Deferred" income is not taxed in the current tax period, but will be taxed eventually:

- Sale of personal residence
- Retirement plan earnings and deposits made to them (IRAs, profit sharing, defined benefit, SEPP, and 401K)
- Growth stock appreciation
- Appreciation in value of real estate
- Installment sales of business or property

"Exempt" income is not taxed:

- Tax-exempt bond interest
- Fifty or 100 percent of social security benefits
- Scholarships
- Tax-shelter income

From this listing it becomes clear that business owners can benefit from a "qualified retirement plan." Any contribution to the plan will reduce taxable income. Earning are not taxed until withdrawn from the plan. Chapter 18 discusses these plans in detail.

In discussing the formula for the 1040 tax return, deductions were mentioned. Deductions are subtractions from income:

The "personal exemption" is a flat amount that can be deducted for each taxpayer and each dependent. The law adjusts exemption amounts for inflation each year.

The "standard deduction" is a flat amount that can be deducted on a tax return if the taxpayer chooses not to itemize deductions, or if the taxpayer does not have enough deductions to permit itemization. It is adjusted for inflation annually.

Alimony is deductible by the payer and taxable income to the recipient. The rules on how the payments are made, and over what period of time, are complicated and are interpreted by the Internal Revenue Service in a strict fashion. Professional advice should be sought to insure that payments are deductible.

Child-support payments are neither deductible by the payer nor taxable to the recipient. Under current law, the custodial parent has the right to deduct the dependent child unless a divorce decree states otherwise, or the custodial parent signs a special Internal Revenue Service form relinquishing the right to the exemption. Each child claimed must have a social security number.

Moving expenses can be deducted if related to the commencement of work in new location. Deductible moving expenses include:
- Travel to the new location
- Transporting possessions
- Pre-move house-hunting trips
- Temporary living expenses for up to 30 days in the new location
- Disposition cost of the old and residence acquisition costs of the new residence (attorney's fees, real estate commissions, and so forth)

Auto mileage can be deducted at a rate of nine cents per mile as part of the travel expenses. There is a complicated distance test. To be allowed the moving expense deduction, a taxpayer must work in the new location for thirty-nine weeks unless moved again because of a new transfer.

Medical expenses are not deductible until they exceed 7.5 percent of adjusted gross income. Prescription drugs are included, over-the-counter remedies are not. Medical insurance and medical transportation are deductible, as are health-care costs not reimbursed by insurance.

State and local income taxes and personal property and real estate taxes are deductible. Sales taxes are not deductible by individuals, but sales taxes on business equipment and vehicles can be written off as the equipment is depreciated.

Whether interest paid can be deducted depends on why the money was borrowed and what asset secures the loan. Interest on first- and second-residence mortgages can be deducted, subject to limits. Interest paid on business mortgages and other business purpose loans is fully deductible.

The consumer-interest deduction which some of us remember from the past has been eliminated since 1991. Thus none of the consumer interest paid is deductible. Consumer interest is interest on such items as credit cards, autos, personal bank loans, or student loans. To the extent that credit cards and autos are used for business, that portion of the interest can be deducted in full on the appropriate business tax return (Schedule C of Form 1040, Form 1120 for corporate returns, and Form 1065 for partnerships).

Charitable contributions continue to be deductible. The value of goods donated to charity and charitable mileage at twelve cents per mile may be deducted.

Miscellaneous deductions have been severely restricted by the new law. They are deductible only to the extent that the expenses exceed 2 percent of the taxpayer's adjusted gross income. Some of the expenses deductible in this category:

- Employee unreimbursed business travel
- Employee unreimbursed auto expenses
- Business subscriptions
- Job-hunting expenses
- Tax preparation and consulting
- Safe-deposit box
- Trustee fees
- Legal expenses related to the production of income
- Uniforms (cost and maintenance)
- Professional dues

Business meals are deductible, but the deduction is limited to 50 percent of the business meal expenses. A business meal is one at which a discussion with a client, patient, colleague, or adviser occurs about something related to the entrepreneur's business. In order for the deduction to be allowed, the following must be recorded (in writing) at the time of each business meal:

- Place
- Date

- Amount spent
- Who was there
- What the business purpose was

Business entertainment expenses are also deductible up to the 50 percent limit. The entertainment must be "quiet" and appropriate. There are rather strict rules defining these words, and attention must be paid to assure qualifications of the deduction.

Deductible out-of-town travel expenses include the cost of travel, lodging, and meals. Detailed records and receipts must be kept.

Child-care credit is the only credit to survive the new law worth mentioning. If child care expenses are paid so that the taxpayer and spouse can attend school or work, a percentage of the expenses can be recovered as a subtraction from taxes due.

Business Income Taxes

A corporation is a taxable entity separate from the owner(s); a sole proprietorship or partnership is not. A corporation files its own tax return (Form 1120 or 1120A, depending on the size of the practice). If a profit is earned in a corporation, the corporation must pay corporate taxes. The remaining profits can then be paid out to shareholders as dividends. Shareholders are taxed on any dividends they receive. Thus, the profits are in effect taxed twice. Normally, this is avoided in a closely held corporation by paying the profits out in the form of salaries to the owner-employee.

As indicated in Chapter 5, corporations may choose between two basic treatments of profit for tax purposes, a "C" or an "S" corporation. A "C" corporation is a taxable entity in and of itself. A stockholder-employee is treated as any other employee, except with respect to qualified retirement plans. Corporate tax rates effective July 1, 1987, are as follows:

Up to $50,000 net income	15%
Over $50,000 to $75,000	25%
Over $75,000	34%

In addition, a surcharge of 5 percent on taxable income over $100,000 is levied until the benefit of the lower rates is phased out. This creates a 39 percent marginal rate on incomes from $100,000 to $335,000.

Notice that a "C" corporation pays only 15 percent tax on the first $50,000 of net income. The example of Dr. Jones earlier in this chapter shows that it doesn't take a lot of income before reaching a 50 percent tax rate as an individual. A common strategy has been to leave up to $50,000 per year in profits in the corporation, paying the lower tax rate available. The law has a section, entitled Accumulated Excess Retained Earnings, intended to avoid long-term abuse of the tax rate differential. The IRS can penalize (an excise penalty tax) excess retained earnings above $150,000 in a corporation. Typically, these excess accumulations are invested in cash, stock, CD's, and the like, and not used for any purpose by the corporation. This investment pattern is a signal to the IRS to investigate for accumulated earnings. The board of directors can create a legitimate business purpose for the accumulation, like saving to buy a building or to fund a corporate buy-sell agreement, to avoid penalties levied under this provision.

An advantage of the corporate business form is that in the beginning of the practice when cash flow is tight, owners may wish to borrow some funds from the corporation instead of paying themselves a salary. This could save money otherwise spent on payroll taxes.

A section of the Internal Revenue Code, new in the 1986 tax law, creates the personal services corporation. This is a corporation that receives income from the services performed by professionals. All health-care providers who incorporate will probably fall under this section of the code. It eliminates the first two steps of the tax tables, thus taxing even one dollar of profit left in the corporation at the 34 percent rate. The message from Uncle Sam seems to be: You are really an individual; we believe you have high income; if you do not submit to the individual tax rate, we will penalize you in this manner.

An "S" corporation is taxed like a sole proprietor, except that the "S" provides some advantages of limited liability and can issue stock. This form could be useful in the early years of a business if losses are incurred. The losses are passed through to the owner's tax return and can be used to shelter other income, for instance, spousal income. The election to be treated as an "S" corporation must be filed with the IRS before it is valid. There are specific rules on when during a tax year the election can be filed. Professional help is probably required to assure correct timing.

A sole proprietor is taxed based on the following formula: Profit or loss is determined by subtracting expenses from revenue. The proprietor must pay both income taxes and self-employment taxes on the profit. This calculation is performed on Schedule C of the proprietor's income tax return. The profit is listed on the front of Form 1040 for income tax purposes, and on Form SE for self-employment taxes. The SE tax is added, on the back of the 1040, to determine the total tax due Uncle Sam. One of the expenses that can be taken on Schedule C is the depreciation expense. (For a definition of depreciation refer to the first section of Chapter 13.) Computers may be depreciated over five years, furniture, equipment, and fixtures can be written off in any of three ways: accelerated depreciation over seven years, or straight-line depreciation over eight years, or expensing up to $17,500 in the first year.

Again the authors wish to point out the importance of up-to-date, current knowledge in this area. Accountants certainly can be expected to do the number crunching for the entrepreneur, but a basic understanding of the concepts and procedures is required to make proper busienss decisions with regard to timing and titling of equipment and property purchases. Decisions such as when to buy or lease are heavily influenced by the tax treatment anticipated. The IRS publications and seminars mentioned earlier in this chapter really are excellent avenues for learning.

If a high tax bracket is expected in the first year or two in business, then one of the two methods that give big deductions early in the life of the equipment (accelerated depreciation or expensing) would probably be more beneficial. If profitability is expected to start slowly and build gradually, the straight-line method might be the optimal choice. To obtain the full depreciation deduction, no more than 40 percent of the total equipment purchases may be made in the final quarter of the tax year.

Automobiles can be depreciated over a five-year period. The taxpayer can use any of the three depreciation methods described earlier, but there is a limit on the amount that can be expensed. This limit is the "luxury automobile" limitation. The limit changes each year with inflation. The car must be used for business purposes more than 50 percent to be eligible to use the "fast" depreciation methods. This percentage must be maintained in future years to avoid depreciation recapture.

The taxpayer has the choice either to use a standard mileage rate per business mile or to track all actual expenses of operating the vehicle. The standard rate is announced by the IRS each year in October; for 1997 it is 31.5 cents per business mile. If the actual-expense approach is chosen, only that portion of expenses that equates to the percentage of business use can be deducted. Actual automobiles costs include:

- Gas and oil
- Car washes
- Insurance
- Repairs and maintenance
- Licenses
- Interest
- Lease payments
- Depreciation

In addition to expense records, the taxpayer must keep a meticulous mileage log to prove to the Internal Revenue Service what percentage of the total miles driven were in business use. This log must be maintained whether the standard mileage rate or actual expense deduction is chosen.

Commercial-use buildings can be written off on a straight-line basis over a 31.5-year period. Land cannot be depreciated, nor can a personal residence. If part of the residence is used for a qualifying in-home office, that part of the residence can be depreciated. In addition, part of the cost of utilities, maintenance, rent, and other costs must be used exclusively for business. In general, an in-home office cannot be claimed if another office, located in a business property, is available.

Summary

Taxes are a rather complex matter. Accountants and tax attorneys spend as much time in professional school, preparing for their position in society, as do physicians. The intent of this chapter is to provide some basic understanding of the terminology and concepts with which every entrepreneur needs to become familiar. Only professionals can make specific applicable law determinations based on the facts of a case. Advice from a qualified tax adviser is indispensable to the business owner.

There are many facets to taxes that have not been discussed in this chapter. Such topics as investment treatment, passive activity losses, or limited partnerships are all well beyond the scope intended here. We stated at the beginning that dealing with taxes is becoming a large part of the entrepreneur's daily activity. The trend over the last four decades has been that taxes have increased at a steeply progressive rate. Nothing can be seen in the future that will reverse this trend.

15

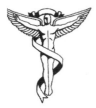 # The Business Plan

Most health-care providers starting a business for the first time have the expectation—the conviction—that, when the business opens its doors, patients will be standing outside waiting. In fact, most entrepreneurs have this feeling at the start. With professionals, however, it seems especially common because of their feelings that they have received the best possible, most up-to-date education and are such fantastic individuals (or so everyone has told them). It is a rude awakening indeed, when the fateful day finally arrives, to discover that no one knows about the new clinic.

PPB, the first three concepts of our system of management, were designed to assist. If followed as explained in Chapter 2, a written business plan will result. If followed correctly, using the concepts of vision, mission, and the others as explained in Chapter 4, a high-quality plan will result. Two examples of business plans and loan proposals that have yielded success (if such is measured by obtaining bank financing for practice startup or purchase) are located in Appendices G and H. In this chapter we will provide some hints that are helpful in the creation of a business plan.

We may have only hinted at it so far, so it is time to be very direct. The process of writing a business plan is long, arduous, frustrating, cyclical, invigorating, and much more. All our positive and negative emotions will come out. Therefore, the authors find it important for the budding entrepreneur to realize that the time spent creating this plan from a simple dream to a completed document is one of the most crucial times in the development of a business owner. Learning happens rapidly during the process. And yes, the process is as important as the result.

The plan's outline is simple to conceive: for each topic dealt with, the approach should be from the broad, fuzzy vision to the objectives, goals, strategies, and action steps that will allow it to become reality. Understand that the vision is an overall view. Specific personnel and functional responsibility areas are needed to attain it. That is where the objective, goals, strategies, and action steps come in. Those allow us to define the road to the destination.

As indicated in Chapter 4, mindset is a strength and a weakness at the same time. It allows us the determination to finish the planning process, while it put blinders on us and forces us to stay on track. Too often, the track is so narrow we overlook obvious hurdles just off to the side. The authors have recommended that the written document be shared with others at various stages of its development. This approach will avoid having the mindset blinders too narrowing, while at the same time giving others a chance to become enthusiastic about the vision. We call these others "advisors." Advisors will be discussed in detail below. Commonly, the most important ones are referred to in the plan document, in the principals section.

Advisors

By using the term advisors, we do not mean to imply that only compensated, highly trained individuals should be considered. The most important characteristic of an advisor is that the entrepreneur will listen to him or her. This indicates that spouses, parents, and friends should be considered in the selection process. Communication between the advisor and the advisee is crucial. We grant that specific business knowledge is an advantage. However, not all decisions to be made in drafting a business plan require business knowledge. To return to the example used in describing planning in Chapter 6, the location decision is much more a personal preference than a business decision.

Once the personal advisors have been selected, it is time to look for qualified professionals. Advisors come in many forms, shapes, and appearances, as well as in a large number of specialties. At a minimum, the starting entrepreneur needs an accountant, an attorney in business and tax law, an insurance counselor, and a banker. Some entrepreneurs find it necessary also to have a successful businessperson.

Assuming we understand the need for advisors, the big question becomes always how and where to find them. The most important consideration in making a choice is that the entrepreneur needs to be comfortable with the individual, to trust the advice being provided, and to be willing to implement it. Each entrepreneur is an individual with a unique personality, and the person who advises the owner of company A may not be the individual who will work well with the owner of company B. This is not to impugn anyone's technical knowledge or personality. Friendship between advisor and advisee is not a necessity; however, respect and trust are.

As a result, the best way to find appropriate advisors is for the entrepreneur to ask friends, acquaintances, colleagues, and competitors about who they use. It is to be expected that if Dr. A and Dr. B are friends, they have certain attitudes and personality traits in common and the consequent likelihood of being able to work with the same individual.

Just because an someone comes highly recommended, is extremely intelligent and knowledgeable, and has a good reputation, is no guarantee that the entrepreneur and the advisor will work well together. The entrepreneur has enough basic knowledge to determine the compatibility level. It is suggested that the entrepreneur spend some time working with the potential advisor prior to actually making the selection, and, if necessary, paying a few hours' worth of fees, in order to arrive at a conclusion as to the comfort, trust, and acceptability of that person for the particular entrepreneur. As with any planning step, more than one potential advisor should probably be considered. Let us discuss the various professionals in some detail.

Accountants

Accountants come with different levels of capabilities, costs, and services provided. The national standard for capability is three letters behind the name of the individual: CPA (Certified Public Accountant). Many accountants who do not have a CPA are highly qualified and extremely capable of providing good advice to the beginning entrepreneur. Fees range from a few hundred dollars per hour when one employs an accountant from one of the Big Six firms, to perhaps as little as $25 an hour for the non-CPA bookkeeping type of accountant in the local rural environment.

The minimum one should expect from an accountant is assistance in creating an adequate bookkeeping system, and in the writing of loan proposals. Assistance with calculations for cash-flow projections and risk analysis, and preparation of tax returns and the calculation of the tax effects of certain anticipated purchases, are also within the capabilities of accountants.

Early inclusion of the accountant in the planning, programming, and budgeting portion of the creation of the business is highly recommended. Some accountants specialize in assisting small, newly created businesses. Obviously it is advantageous for the new entrepreneur to find an accountant of this variety. Besides assisting in the initial cash-flow and risk analysis and the determination of the capital and working capital budgets, the accountant should be capable of creating a usable bookkeeping system for the entrepreneur.

If the entrepreneur has chosen to utilize an automated office approach right from the start and has selected an office management software package, making the accountant aware of this decision and bringing the accountant up to date on the software program and its capabilities will save tremendous amounts of time later.

The accountant's function is to generate financial statements for the business owner to review, enabling him or her to determine the progress of the business. These statements are sometimes given to friendly outsiders; bankers in particular are interested in seeing financial statements on a regular basis. Although many accountants attempt to save client fees by not generating financial statements more frequently than annually, it is suggested that, in order to work the control function of PPBIC appropriately, statements be drafted at least quarterly. A major function of the accountant is to supervise the financial record and reporting system and to assist in recognizing the tax consequences of any action of the entrepreneur. Let it be clearly understood that business decisions should not be made solely on the basis of tax effect, but rather on the basis of business or economic common sense. Tax effect, however, may have a large influence on the approach implemented for a given situation.

Lawyers

The lawyer is an advisor who should be involved from the inception, in fact, the preinception of the business. The appropriate attorney with business and tax knowledge will be able to assist in reviewing real estate leases, equipment leases, the form of business chosen, and employment agreements, as well as many other business functions.

Some business attorneys have a tendency to dot every *i* and cross every *t*, thus slowing down the decision-making process. While precision is important, there is an appropriate time and place for it. Therefore, it should be remembered that with the attorney, as with all advisers, the entrepreneur is in charge of the relationship. It is the prerogative of the business owner to decide what will be done. It is the function of the attorney to counsel the entrepreneur on the legal effects of the decision to be made. Finally, the attorney's function is to assist the entrepreneur in drafting agreements which may have legal consequences. Today attorneys are capable of drafting legal instruments in English, rather than in Philadelphia legalese. For the benefit of all parties concerned, the entrepreneur should insist on clear language in all agreements.

The right attorney, who should be visited on a regular basis by the entrepreneur, will also be able to assist the entrepreneur in such areas as long-term financial planning and estate and tax planning. Estate planning can be as simple as the drafting and execution of a will, or it may be as complex as a will and a number of trusts, a number of gifting documents, and other highly technical and involved instruments.

Like every other advisor, the attorney should be willing to acknowledge the limit of his or her capabilities and to refer the entrepreneur to a more appropriate counselor when necessary.

Insurance Counselors

Insurance counselors may be deemed hard to find, as most insurance people are salespeople. The general population tends to react adversely toward salespeople, and many highly qualified and professional insurance counselors walk around under a wide variety of titles. Agent, salesperson, account executive, and account manager are all popular today. Some insurance people present themselves as financial planners, which only adds to the confusion.

A knowledgeable insurance person can assure the entrepreneur of the proper coverages for property, casualty, life, health, and pension insurance. The right individual should be willing to survey the market for the appropriate product and price. This last statement may display a bias to independent insurance people, as they have access to a variety of insurance carriers. Frequently, direct writing agents are as capable as independents, but will need to refer to a salesperson with another company for those coverages their employers cannot provide in an adequate manner.

Whether the entrepreneur chooses to work with one independent agent or with a number of insurance salespeople is immaterial, as long as someone is in charge of supervising the entire risk-management picture.

Bankers

It is incumbent upon the entrepreneur to develop a relationship with a banker over time so that the banker becomes a valued advisor instead of an unfriendly critic.

Relationships with bankers are developed by being oneself and truthful. Performing as promised by making payments on time develops trust on the part of the banker in the statements of the entrepreneur. Experience has shown that bankers will work with entrepreneurs if kept fully informed of the problems faced by the business. Relationship problems arise when the entrepreneur is not willing to communicate about unanticipated financial difficulties he or she encounters. No promise is being made here that bankers will have opened purses at all times. If, however, true temporary setbacks occur, most bankers, when fully informed, will assist the entrepreneur by facilitating changes in the loan repayment schedule.

Most professionals coming out of school today do so with large student loans. This makes it difficult for bankers to lend money for a new clinic. No one likes to walk up to a stranger to ask to borrow money. The banker relationship starts, as a result, in the most difficult of circumstances for both parties. Only goodwill and open communication can overcome this obstacle.

Business Owners

Colleagues, especially those with more experience, can be of tremendous assistance to anyone starting a career. The smart entrepreneur will, therefore, spend large amounts of time picking the brains of those people who have had to face the same problems and questions. Assuming mutual respect, most business owners are more than willing to discuss their approach to running a business. Only when immediate, direct competition is involved are you likely to observe any reluctance to share knowledge.

An excellent device for utilizing the knowledge and experience of successful business owners is the informal board of directors. A board of directors can be used whether or not the business form requires it. The following approach is suggested: Find a small number of business owners in different fields of endeavor; determine your comfort level with and trust in these people; invite those who can contribute to your success to join the board of directors; act, with relation to your board, as if it were a formalized structure.

It may be necessary to formalize your relationship with the board of directors to the extent that regular meetings are held. Compensation may have to be paid, although most business owners receive enough in the form of the ego-income that results from assisting a colleague. The most important factor is the attitude of the entrepreneur. A true desire to learn and receive assistance will almost always be responded to as requested. Our best advice is to utilize the members of the board of directors as resource persons, and to allow them to have decision-making powers in the policy-setting of the business.

A pleasant side benefit of the above approach is that the entrepreneur is no longer the sole responsible individual. As a result, the loneliness of having to make all decisions, without available support and understanding, has been alleviated.

The Business Plan

With all the help indicated above, some thoughts and ideas will soon appear on paper. If it is still not quite clear what the business plan consists of, the confusion may result from the fact that a business plan is really a personal document. No two are alike. In order to alleviate concern, we present the following list:

- Cash-flow projections and pro formas
- Marketing plan (who, what, when, how)
- Business legal structure
- Capital asset structure (purchase versus lease)
- Financial plan (startup, capital, working capital)

- Real estate lease (enlargement, other tenants, sublease, bailout)
- Professional review (accountant, lawyer, banker, business manager)
- Board of directors
- Advertising program (yellow pages, billboards, newspapers, coupons, direct mail, TV, radio)
- Personnel (if any) to be hired

This list is not complete, and every individual will have a few items to add. It is intended only as a guide to the basic topics to be included. As can be clearly seen, this step-by-step approach will require continual climbing back up the ladder in order to revise some of the "completed" steps. It is true that "a manager's job is never finished," and PPIBC is a continuous activity.

To offer an approach slightly different from the one employed to generate the documents of Appendices H and G, the following business plan outline might develop some beneficial thoughts in the reader:

A. Business data
 1. Business name
 2. Business address
 3. Business structure
 4. What chiropractic is (a brief explanation from broad to specific)

B. Personal profile (a narrative description, not a résumé)
 1. Name and position in the business (including an indication of full- or part-time)
 2. Previous business and employment experiences relative to this venture
 3. Volunteer work experiences
 4. Education
 5. Extracurricular activities
 6. Recreational activities

C. Business Plan Summary
 1. Location and why it was selected
 2. Patient base (Where will they come from? Marketing plan.)
 3. Community interest (What civic groups will you join? Will you be living there?)
 4. Anticipated opening date and hours the office will be open (including twenty-four-hour call arrangements)

    5. Type of advertisement (opening notice to papers, brochures, or flyers)

    6. Graph projections of patient volume with new-patient growth over one year, three years, and five years

    7. Office staff

    8. Planned equipment additions

D. Projections

    1. Business projections

    2. Cash-flow projections

    3. Pro forma income statements and balance sheet

E. Loan request sheet

F. Personal financial statement (on the bank's requisite forms.)

16

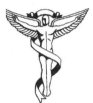 **Getting the Money You Need**

After you decide on the location for your practice, you must arrange to lease or buy the building. If you are buying an existing practice, set up the terms, get prices for equipment, decorating, insurance, supplies, utilities, and staff salaries. Estimate your living expenses for the time period calculated as necessary in the cash-flow projections. All of this is in preparation for financing.

There are several sources to investigate when financing your practice. Banks are the most likely source of financing. Most doctors coming out of school already have large student loans. Several rejections may occur before someone responds positively, but keep trying.

Bankers

Assets, current debt, business plan, cash-flow projections, bank repayment, and collateral are examined by bankers in loan proposals. Bankers make lending decisions based on two factors: the financial prospects of the business and the character of the borrower. The concern of the bank is, Will we be paid on time? Be prepared before you talk with your banker. A banker looks at the following:

- Itemized projection of expenses and revenue
- Commitment to reinvest cash flow in building the practice

- Loan payback arrangements in case of business failure (collateral)
- Current liabilities and their repayment arrangements
- Interest and involvement in the community

The logical assumption for everyone starting a business is that the friendly local banker will receive prospective borrowers with open arms and checkbook. After all, we can believe advertisements, can't we? Well, reality has been called the school of hard knocks, and with good reason. There are right and wrong ways to apply for a loan. The right way is the one that leads to the issuance of a check to the entrepreneur in return for the signing of a note. It is difficult to predict what will or will not work with bankers.

Loan Proposals

Loan proposals come in various shapes and forms. While most commonly a loan proposal consist of the business plan (see Chapter 15) to which one sheet (the loan request) is added, there is no way of predicting the most effective shape and form. However, simplicity and appropriate brevity appear to be the common themes. Bankers tell us that they are pressed for time, and presentation of a small book is probably not the smartest thing to do, assuming one wishes to have a positive response to the effort. The major factor for success appears to be organization of the material and a display of understanding of the requirements of running a successful business. Available collateral and a cosigner's willingness to support the starting entrepreneur are obviously assisting factors. This fact notwithstanding, many graduating physicians with negative net worth, no collateral, and no available cosigners have been successful in obtaining loans. A loan proposal should be short and well organized, of neat and professional appearance. Many entrepreneurs, when applying for a loan, use the old presenter's technique of writing a rather short presentation (six to ten pages) which is then followed by a long, thick series of appendices containing all possible details. Sometimes these appendices are offered in a separate binding, to make it clear to the banker that there really is not all that much reading material.

Cash-flow projections for the first three years of operation are probably required; pro forma balance sheets and projected income statements may be welcomed by the banker. These papers have a rather standard format. Normally, the figures for the first year are summarized by quarter, and the second- and third-year figures are given on an annual basis. All this is normally already included in the business plan (which became the loan proposal, remember?).

The loan request sheet states the total amount which is to be borrowed, and provides an indication of the desired terms of the loan. It might be wise to request a particular split between term loan and working capital line of credit, if a separation is desired. If any collateral or cosigners will be available, that should be stated as well. If a principal repayment moratorium will be requested, this should be indicated. Below the request, indicate how the moneys borrowed will be used. If a term loan is requested, usage of funds should be outlined in summarized form. The following is a suggested format:

1.	Equipment to be purchased	$XXXXXX
2.	Leasehold improvements	$YYYYYY
3.	Start-up expenses (including initial office supplies and rent deposit)	$ZZZZZZZ
4.	Total	$AAAAAA

The request for a working capital line of credit can be supported by a statement, referring to the cash-flow projections, which shows the maximum deficit to be anticipated, the time in the operation of the business for which this deficit low point is projected, and the speed with which recovery from the deficit is expected.

A complete list of equipment, solidly quoted for price and delivery, and the detailed cash-flow projections should probably not be included. If the entrepreneur has a strong desire to let the banker know, those may be included as an appendix. When anticipating your personal financial needs for the year, estimate the least amount needed to live on (suggestion: figure on what your living expenses were as a student).

Please note that no references from professors, friends, ministers, associates, or peers are included above. Instead, a statement that references are available on request should be on the business and personal information sheet. Should the banker actually read this section of the proposal and request references, ask about the specific information desired from each reference. This process will allow the entrepreneur to match sources with the specific information needed.

One source of funds is preferable to spreading the business debt over many entities. With multiple loans, juggling payments as cash flow allows becomes a problem. It is easier to remember to pay the bank a large amount each month than to remember a number of smaller payments to various lenders and leasing companies.

The preferred loan structure is a term loan for the equipment and startup cost, and a line of credit for working capital needs. The total of these two loans rarely is less than $35,000 for a "from scratch" practice; $50,000 to $70,000 is not unusual. Monthly payments on those amounts will range from $500 to $1,500 or more per month. Realistic planning and expectations before opening a practice will reduce unwelcome stress during the crucial Valley of Death period.

If you are not knowledgeable about accounting (this is not unusual), retain an accountant. His or her professional knowledge may increase your chances of receiving a loan and save you enough money to pay for the accounting services you've received.

Submitting the Proposal

Bankers like to know with whom they are doing business. It is therefore suggested that a personal visit to the banker to discuss the possibility of borrowing, leaving the loan proposal behind, will yield you better results than the mass-mailing approach. You can easily arrange a personal visit (by appointment) with the most senior loan officer. The appointment should follow a specific time schedule controlled by you. Following a warmup and get-acquainted period, the purpose of the visit is at hand, and you should provide the banker a general verbal description of the loan request. You should now gauge the banker's initial reaction in order to determine whether or not the discussion should continue. Assuming a positive reception at this point, offer the loan proposal, and provide the banker an opportunity for a quick review. When you hand over the paperwork it might be wise to make a statement such as, "Here is what I have put together. All of the information included is supported by detailed paperwork, which I will be delighted to provide if you desire." This approach allows the banker the flexibility of asking you those questions and for that information which will assist him or her in determining the viability of a lending decision.

A Quick Review of Current Banking Practices

A decade ago, prior to the large and rapid increases in interest rates, banks were in the habit of lending money through what are called term loans. In this kind of loan money is lent for a specific period of time, to be repaid in monthly payments consisting of principal and interest. During the early 1980s banks were in the unpleasant position of having to pay high interest rates in order to acquire deposits, while much of their asset base was lent out in long-term, relatively low-interest-rate loans. The savings and loan defaults and bankruptcies of the late 1980s have created even more concern about interest rate flexibility on long-term loans. As a result, banks have changed their way of doing business. Currently a typical loan is on a relatively short-term note, varying from three months to three years, at a fixed or floating interest rate. The floating interest rate is calculated using a formula. For example, most loans are at a certain percentage over prime. Prime is an artificial interest rate established by large money-center banks and supposedly available only to their best commercial customers. Most starting entrepreneurs can borrow at rates varying between 1 and 2.5 percent over prime.

Whether a loan has a floating prime-plus rate or a fixed interest rate for the term of the note, normally the amount borrowed is such that it cannot be repaid in reasonably attainable monthly installments over the short term; therefore, bankers are willing to amortize loans over periods longer than the supporting note, resulting in a lump sum amount due at the end. Bankers anticipate refinancing this amount remaining at the end of the note. It is highly recommended that during the initial discussion you request a commitment to such refinancing. Bankers are wary of providing such a commitment on paper to the starting entrepreneur. However, a verbal or written commitment should be obtainable, assuming loan payments are made as currently being discussed.

The danger of this approach, from the entrepreneur's point of view, is that it is perfectly possible at the end of, say, two years, that $30,000 still remains of the loan when the note becomes due. Should the entrepreneur's situation, or the general economic situation have changed, the bank may not be willing to refinance this balance, at which point the entrepreneur has the unpleasant task of attempting to refinance it elsewhere. It's back to square one, as if starting the practice all over. If payments on the loan have been made as originally projected, however, the entrepreneur is now in a more advantageous position to provide a new banker with a track record of a few years' operation. The main reason for bankers' working with these short-term notes is to provide, from time to time, the opportunity to adjust the interest rates being earned on outstanding loans. It is not the banker's intention to negate promises made on the total financing periods.

A humorous look at what can transpire in a banker's office will introduce some concepts. Let us for a moment imagine ourselves as the banker. Here comes the professional school graduate, who sits down in the easy chair in our office, without having arranged for an appointment to see us, and who says something like, "Say, I need some money, and I figured you will give it to me." Now, most of us in the role of banker would manage to hide our irritation with this person and feign interest, even if our lunch is being postponed. A little questioning will reveal that the individual (whom we shall hereafter call A) has recently graduated from PDQ professional school, which he states is the best, most progressive in its profession, and would like to start practice in our town. He has no idea where in town he will hang his hat. He states that we can safely lend him $125,000, because in his first year he figures to make two or three times that much. After all, he graduated eighty-fifth out of his class of 110, and everyone above him has already made at least that much. He just needed a few months to recuperate from the last few years of high-intensity study.

Let us assume further that there is something we cannot define about A that stops us from terminating the discussion at this time. After a difficult discussion about such matters as his assets, pro forma, and working capital needs, (he clearly never read chapter 13), we arrive at the understanding that today he is between $60,000 and $65,000 in debt, that he just last month married a young woman in the class behind him. He says, "The family that works together, stays together," and he intends to prove it. He says that he will pay the loan back in no time at all, and that $48,000 of it is necessary for that beautiful Mercedes he saw on the lot down the street.

To really finish this story off correctly, we must assume that we, the banker, lend the money, and that A squanders it but in spite of himself manages to build a successful practice. The close cooperation in the offices does not work, he divorces his wife. He returns to his school for homecoming some years later and spends a few moments in the business and practice management class. He tells the students to be blunt and demanding when asking for loan money. It worked for him; it will work for them. He is not aware, and probably never will be, that shortly after he left our (the banker's) office his grandfather called us. Grandpa has enough cash in our bank to buy the bank, should he want to.

The conversation between us, the banker, and Grandpa went something like this: "This is Grandpa Deeppockets. My grandson said he would stop by to see you today. I want you to give him whatever he asks for, but do not let him know that I will guarantee the loan. He needs a success on his own, so let him think that he convinces you. Send me whatever papers I need to sign to make sure you have adequate collateral guarantee." No wonder we wrote a check for $125,000 and did not care if we ever saw our fine physician again. This vignette displays (with a modicum of sarcasm) all concepts and concerns discussed so far in this chapter. Assets, current debts, business plan, cash-flow projections, personal needs, payback, and collateral are all present.

Other Sources

It is always a possibility that commercial banks, despite many attempts by the entrepreneur to secure loans, will be unwilling to lend money for the venture being proposed. There are other sources of financing available. Other options include savings passbook loans, cash value of life insurance policies, mortgages or second mortgages, collateral loans, relatives/ friends, a silent partner, and small business loans. Among them the Small Business Administration (SBA) has a direct lending program for professionals starting a practice. The requirements are a denial of loan request by at least two commercial banks, submission of an SBA loan request document (obtainable from the local SBA office), and approval of the loan by the Small Business Administration. Frequently the total funds available to the SBA for this sort of lending purpose are limited. The entrepreneur, therefore, needs to be prepared to wait as much as eighteen months for the moneys requested, even assuming he or she received an initial positive response from the SBA.

In recent years, the SBA has made "low doc loans" available through local banks. Low doc refers to the amount of documentation the borrower and the bank must submit to the SBA. These loans are applied for through, and with the assistance of, the bank and are frequently approved or declined in less then a week. As the bank carries major responsibility (the SBA acts as guarantor for the borrower up to a stated percentage of the balance) for the loan, the only approach to this kind of loan is through the banker. Most bankers do not wish to be bothered with the paperwork for a loan of less then $100,000, so be prepared to increase your loan request and, of course, to justify the increased amount. A number of our clients have successfully accomplished this. The loan is a line of credit for the first year, at the end of which any remaining available funds are "pulled" and a savings account at the bank is opened with that money. This money is left to sit there until the entrepreneur clearly has made the turn in the Valley of Death. At that point a large principal payment is made on the loan. All in all, a very satisfactory manner of doing business (win-win-win) for all concerned: the chiropractor, the banker, and the SBA.

Families and friends are excellent sources of capital for starting a venture. Friends in this case can certainly include the seller of the practice, should that be the situation. In dealing with friends and family, a business approach should be taken with regard to the transaction. This means that a note is signed, a reasonable near-market interest rate negotiated, and an amortization schedule drafted. There are multiple reasons for this suggestion, among them psychological factors inherent in doing business with family and friends. In addition, from the lender's point of view, there are income tax reasons. While certainly not the overriding factor, those ought to be considered and honored by the entrepreneur.

An option available to many starting entrepreneurs is to rent or lease equipment. There are two types of lease currently used in the financial markets. One we shall call the operational lease; it is the true lease form and can be compared to renting an apartment for living space or an office location for the practice. It means there will never be ownership of the equipment; no down payment is required; there is a monthly payment made for usage of equipment. For the lessee there are none of the tax benefits normally attached to ownership; all tax benefits accrue to the lessor. From an income-tax point of view the operational lease payments should be totally tax-deductible to the entrepreneur. All repair and maintenance charges are typically the responsibility of the lessor; occasionally these are negotiated to be the responsibility of the lessee. The second form of lease is the financial lease. This is actually a form of purchase of the equipment, utilizing the installment method. A down payment is required up front; monthly payments are made; some tax benefits such as partial depreciation may come to the lessee; and a tail-end purchase clause may be included. This approach is used by many equipment manufacturers, including car manufacturers. The "open-ended" car lease is a perfect example of a financial lease. The financial lease is actually similar to borrowing money in order to purchase the equipment, even though the lease does not require the purchase of that equipment at the end of the term. The advantage of leasing over purchasing with borrowed money is that there is a lower up-front cash requirement. Occasionally, as a result of the desire of the manufacturer to sell the equipment, a lower interest rate can be negotiated. Besides the obvious financial advantages, leasing allows the entrepreneur to use and become acquainted with the equipment prior to making the purchase decision.

Many finance companies are willing, against appropriate collateral, to lend money for a large variety of purposes. Their loans commonly carry an interest rate higher than that available from banks or leasing companies, but these may be the only organizations willing to make money available to the starting entrepreneur. Citicorp, Commercial Credit Corporation, Beneficial Finance, and Dial Finance, among others, are examples of this type of organization. Frequently, these organizations are willing to lend money for specific purposes, such as the purchase of office furniture or x-ray equipment or leasehold improvements. They normally desire to have the purchased equipment as collateral. The length of the loan is rather short (no more than three to five years). In recent years these finance companies have withdrawn from the commercial market and now lend money only to individuals. Being incorporated will hinder the entrepreneur in working with this kind of organization.

There also exists the "spousal sponsorship." The spouse is employed outside the practice in a suitable position and earns an income, hopefully adequate to financially support the family. This is often the best way to start a professional office. The income provided by the spouse assures that no money has to be taken out of the business for living expenses, and therefore increases the chances of survival and ultimate success of the practice.

Purchasing a Home/Office Combination

In certain parts of the country, especially outside the larger metropolitan areas, many professionals can practice in offices located in their residences. There are advantages and disadvantages from financial, tax, and psychological points of view. If this approach appeals to the beginning entrepreneur, some soul-searching is required prior to implementation. Some people are quite capable of rising in the morning, having breakfast with the family, and walking through a door into a business establishment. Others will fall into the trap of never really leaving the house. They will be more interested in dealing with the family situation, in taking care of the normal family emergencies, in caring for the children, than in attempting to run a professional office. Sometimes all the correct habits and desires exist in the entrepreneur, but the spouse has trouble separating family and business roles at certain times, and as a result creates a conflict of interest in the business owner (frequently without realization by either spouse of what is happening). Self-knowledge, discipline, and recognition of the spouse's capabilities and attitude are extremely important if the decision is made to operate in a home/office environment.

Tax law imposes a number of restrictive requirements on the home/office combination. If these requirements are met, some tax advantages become available. An accountant can explain in detail the requirements imposed by the Internal Revenue Service. As a general rule, in order to receive tax benefits from an office at home, the arrangement has to be such that the office will not be used for any residential purposes. In addition, it must be the primary business location of the entrepreneur. It is highly recommended that a qualified accountant or tax attorney be involved from the inception of the home/office combination.

From a financial point of view, such a combination may be easier to acquire than any other approach to starting a business. The real estate being purchased will generally qualify as collateral for a loan which in reality is obtained to start the business. It becomes impossible to distinguish between use of the money for real estate investment and use for starting the business, and banks and savings and loans are delighted to lend money for real estate acquisition.

The entrepreneur needs to realize that the value of real estate is affected by the use of that real estate. It may therefore be wiser to purchase an existing home/office residence rather than to remodel a house into a combination. If the remodeling is extensive, there is the danger of creating a special-use residence which may have a reduced market value because of the small number of people interested in that type of arrangement.

Part Five

Now That
You Are Open

17

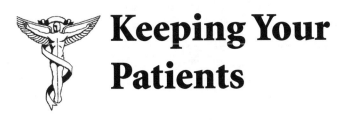 # Keeping Your Patients

Chiropractors are weird, at least when compared to the general population. Chiropractors are very aware of the value of preventative health care, they receive adjustments early and often. In addition, chiropractors receive their care for free. They're weird!

Promoting Wellness
Many young practitioners do not realize that the average American does not have the same understanding of the body's functioning and mechanics as they do. They find it hard to believe that money concerns may influence a person's decisions on the frequency and kind of care desired. Two young (new) practitioners reported earlier this year, "People don't care about their health and they certainly don't want to spend money on it. How come you never told us that in class?" When reminded that this author frequently says just those things, and situational recall was assisted, they acknowledged that they had heard those statements, but did not understand them.

The moral of all this is that the American population needs to be educated with regard to proper health care. America—in fact much of the Western world—is an allopathic environment. Symptomatic relief (doc in the pill) is the known health-care approach (It is scary in this regard to contemplate how many chiropractors and students really have an allopathic approach to life themselves). "Yeah, yeah, Doc, I hear you, just fix my back, it hurts," is a common reaction of patients who are being addressed on the topic of a change in lifestyle. We want instant relief; we live in a microwave society; everything must be done instantaneously. Changing the mindset of people takes time and repeated effort. Chiropractic is the number one preventative health-care profession in the world. We believe that it is high time that chiropractors start spreading the word. As we stated in the preface, the world appears ready to receive the message. Let's do the hard work of educating our patients to improve the health condition of the general population.

Our friends Bill Esteb and Dr. Rob Jackson, of Back Talk Systems, Inc., do a superb job of presenting the necessary messages in a manner understandable to everyone. Other firms also have fine materials and presentations. It behooves the chiropractor to pay attention to these folk and to learn how to communicate effectively with the general public. As the Duke of York (famed of the song) discovered, converting one individual at the time and initiating a chain reaction is a very speedy way to develop an army of 10,000. We do not wish to copy our colleagues mentioned, but feel the need to present some of our thoughts on the topic of promoting wellness. We have learned from past experiences, that the process of educating the patient is a systematic, Chinese water torture treatment process (drip, drip, drip; repeat, repeat, repeat). The cycle is simple: consultation to establish personal communication, exam and studies to determine the causes of the current condition and comorbidity factors, report of findings to provide the education and information necessary for the patient to make informed decisions, care for the condition with a constant reminder of the objective of good health as the patient expresses it, continued education through all phases of care resulting in a life-long chiropractic patient.

Prevention, wellness, holistic: these are words chiropractic has been promoting since its creation, yet for many people these are new concepts. The growth of health awareness and the desire to control one's own body have brought the philosophy of chiropractic to the forefront. Patients seek chiropractic care for the immediate relief of pain or correction of health problems. A logical concomitant should be the introduction of the concepts of wellness and prevention. Holistic medicine is defined by Webster as "treatment of the whole organism, not just the symptoms of a disease."

Treating the whole organism is achieved by creating an atmosphere in the organism (mind and body) promoting wellness, the state of a high level of health. It is a conscious effort, mentally and physically, to eat right, to exercise, to deal effectively with stress, and to avoid foreign chemicals in the system. The lack of wellness may be characterized by any of the following:

- A lack of energy and vitality
- Looking and feeling "out of shape"
- Difficulty coping with daily pressures
- Nagging aches and pains
- Overweight or underweight
- Shortness of breath
- Frequent minor illness
- Loss of muscle tone
- Persistent lower-back pain
- Diminished work performance
- Difficulty concentrating
- More frequent emotional upsets
- Lowered endurance
- Limited flexibility

We are living in a society that is acknowledging the wellness concept. A conscious effort is being made by many to prevent disease instead of waiting for it. In her October 1982 article in *Psychology Today,* "Wellness Is All," Carin Rubenstein writes that respondents to a survey felt that personal health is one of the few remaining safe investments. Factors contributing to poor health include stress, negative emotional responses, lack of exercise, and poor diet. Many respondents supported the holistic approach that the mind influences forces of, and in, the body. People are listening to their bodies, watching for signals of illness or trouble. Rubenstein points out that physical health is a person's last arena of personal control, something all of us can influence. It seems that a desire for good health increases with age, education, and income security, while diseases such as infections, ulcers, and heart problems decrease. Health is a measure of both physical and psychological well-being. By controlling stress in our lives, controlling our diet, sleep, and exercise regimen, we are bringing our bodies to a state of good physical health. By directing our energies into positive thinking and controlling our physical world we avail ourselves of positive psychological energies. Physical control is threatened by outside factors: bacteria, viruses, and toxic environmental agents. These are physical limits that must be acknowledged, and properly dealt with. Through the conscious effort to control and improve our environment, and through positive thinking, through diet and exercise, we as a population are promoting wellness.

Chiropractic is a healing science based on the premise that good health depends upon a normally functioning nervous system. In a survey conducted by the National Research Corporation in the mid-1980s and published by *Modern Health Care* in the April 1985 issue, at least 50 percent of the population acknowledged an interest in wellness and health education. Chiropractors have the wellness concept as a basic part of their professional philosophy. Therefore, they have the prerequisites to assist the patient in changing attitudes and developing health habits.

Specific Steps in Promoting Wellness

There are many things that you can do to promote and improve your patients' health. By encouraging them to pay attention to their bodies through regular exercise, good nutrition, and other preventative maintenance, you will educate them to have a holistic attitude toward their health, thereby promoting their overall wellness.

Exercise

The value of muscle strengthening and improved joint motion rehabilitation programs is understood by us. These exercises have been tested with successful results. Patients need to be made aware of the value of exercise and be encouraged to find their own comfort zone for including it in their lifestyle.

Nutrition

A well-balanced diet is necessary for proper functioning of the body. Through the encouragement of a sensible, well-balanced diet, doctors can support the change in philosophy to preventative health care.

Preventative Maintenance Care

In part, the wellness concept should include a program designed for each patient to maintain his or her health. The stresses of life influence the functioning of the body. Through routine adjustments, chiropractic promotes preventative health care by decreasing nerve interference.

Educational Materials

An effective way to promote wellness is to distribute regular educational letters, pamphlets, and booklets to patients. Design or purchase those that reflect the personal philosophy and style of the practice. Patients who have experienced the positive results of chiropractic care, and have been educated along the way, become excellent referral sources.

Proper professional behavior and documentation is crucial in building the trust and confidence required to allow the patient to accept the educational and informational messages we deliver. As the soil must be prepared and fertilized for the plant seed to germinate into a beautiful flowering plant, so the human mind must be prepared for the seed of education. All parts of the job must be congruent with, and supportive of, the whole. Some thoughts on the paperwork and protocols are therefore in order.

Patient Exams

Know as much as you can about your patient, from his or her lifestyle to the specific complaints that brought your patient into the office. By documenting everything you learn, you will always have a point of refrence to fall back on as you make future decisions concerning your patient's well-being.

Documentation

From the time the patient enters the office and progresses through each level of evaluation, sound documentation is a necessity. The process starts with the consultation and continues through the exam, x-ray, report of findings, and the adjustments. Accurate notes must be taken. A documentation procedure referred to as SOAP notes is used by all the health sciences and is well suited for chiropractic office visits:

S: subjective (patient complaints)
O: objective (executed findings such as x-ray, exam, lab, appearance of genetic handicaps, palpation)
A: assessment (impression)
P: plan (course of action)

Establish with each visit how the patient felt after the last visit, how he or she feels now, and when the change occurred, if any. Each visit, recheck for positive (+) findings, especially severe ones. Note if there is immediate relief. SOAP notes follow the subluxation listings with each visit. A good reference for insurance submission guidelines, and a good source of pertinent information for office protocols, is *The Chiropractic Manual, Second Edition,* originally published by the Ohio State Chiropractic Association in 1990.

The Initial Consultation

The consultation is the first exposure the patient has to the practitioner and the office. The doctor's effectiveness in dealing with people is an important factor in the return to health of the patient. Use of nonverbal communication: eye contact, facial expression, tone of voice, vocal variety, and body posture has been found to have a positive influence on the speed of patient recovery. Interview the patient in a nonthreatening environment. Many patients are not sure what a chiropractor does when they come into the office for the first time as new patients. A strange looking table or model spine as an initial introduction to chiropractic may make a new patient hesitant. As we have become used to seeing them over time, the patient needs the same opportunity for slow, quiet, calm, confidence-building in the tools of the profession. The atmosphere should be comfortable and warm, friendly, and supportive. Although there will be times when the office is busy and jumping, do not rush the patient. The consultation needs to be scripted, the doctor a superb actor who really lives the part. Most people retain only a small percentage of what they hear, especially if they don't feel well. In each conversation, during followup visits, it will be necessary to repeat and reinforce the concepts presented during the consultation. Developing good rapport with the patient is the first step in education. The consultation is the foundation on which the entire process is built.

Exams

After the initial consultation, escort the patient to the exam room. By this time the development of patient-doctor rapport has started. Explain to the patient what to expect through the course of the visit, that is, the exam, x-rays, the recommendation for initiating care, and the expectation of compliance. Have an assistant available to help the patient, explaining what the patient is to do (such as undressing and putting on a gown). Develop a new-patient protocol and stick to it. The first priority is to make the patient feel at ease. Speak slowly and clearly; let the patient know what is being done. Eye contact and touching are taken by most people as a sign of concern for the patient. Patients may not be in a good mood; pain overrides even the most gracious of personalities. Guide the patient through the exam efficiently and with as little distress as possible. In order to achieve the diagnostic results needed, pain may have to be elicited on rare occasions. Explain the procedure before performing it and support the patient emotionally throughout the exam.

After the exam, take necessary x-rays and perform lab studies, schedule a return appointment, perform the adjustment or palliative adjunct therapy as indicated.

Interim Exams
Interim exams (re-exams or updates) are completed as part of a progressive study of the patient. These exams may be performed for a variety of reasons as identified by the physician. The customary interim exam is scheduled when the patient is released from each phase of care. This typically happens between the 10th and 15th visit, and again later when the phase changes to preventative maintenance care. Each patient response to treatment varies, therefore the time frame will vary. Other reasons for interim exams include acute change in status (exacerbation of symptoms), prolonged status of a patient's symptoms without change, a requirement to prove "medical necessity" by the third-party payor, planned change in level of activity, or frequency of care. The frequency of the interim exams in these cases is based upon need as determined by the physician.

Experience suggests that vital signs should be checked during each visit on all hypertensive patients, and once per month on the elderly. This is a valuable service to offer to all patients and may indicate changes in the patient's health. Patients with angina, pacemakers, or cardiac patients of any type, need to have the apical pulse taken in addition to the regular vitals.

In current practice, the recording of orthopedic findings on the exam has shifted away from positives (+) and negatives (-) toward the documentation of actual symptoms. For example, foramina compression, right lateral: instead of simply noting a "+" write out "sharp pain to lateral elbow of R arm." With this type of documentation, the examiner can, at a later date, recheck the test and make a comparative analysis ("second test, foramina compression, right lateral: 'burning' to lateral elbow of R arm"). Keep documentation practices current with the best practices in the profession. Regular continuing education of the chiropractor will avoid embarrassing outdated procedures.

Athletic and Industrial Exams

A service which many chiropractors provide is the athletic, school, or industrial physical. Many times the chiropractor is the only physician a family may see in months. In addition, such physical exams offer convenience for the family, and may be given at lower expense to the patient than other exams. Chiropractors are not only capable of performing the basic physical, they can also perform specialized orthopedic and neurological studies. Maintaining a record of the exam may provide a base-line of information should the patient be injured during the activity for which the exam was performed. In the case of school or sports exams for minors, it is imperative that the parent or guardian complete and sign the appropriate part of the form.

Reports of Findings

Develop a report of findings (ROF) that educates patients enough to understand what their care will involve. Patients need to acknowledge and agree to their need for care. Patients will remember only part of what has been presented. Be direct and to the point about the problem. Let patients know what stage of the Vertebral Subluxation Complex was observed, what it means, and what the recommendation for care is. Be certain to provide full and fair disclosure of possible treatment options and risks. Explain the likely result if treatment is not received. Remember that scaring patients into consenting to treatment is not only inappropriate, it is unethical, may be unprofessional, and typically leads to dissatisfied patients.

The report of findings can be held in a formal setting such as the consultation office, or in the treatment or exam room. Develop a style that is comfortable for patients, speak in plain English, not chiropractese, and solicit as many questions as possible. Questions from patients indicate interest in the topic and provide the feedback needed to assure proper understanding of the information and education. Allow patients time to consider what was reported and to reach necessary decisions.

Written Reports

You will want to have solid, well-organized documentation of your patient's history. Frequently third party payor's will request written reports.

Initial Reports

Initial reports are concise overview reports concerning the patient's present diagnosis, history, and treatment plan. They are usually requested by insurance companies or attorneys in the early stage of a patient's treatment. These reports should be kept brief. Initial reports serve to show medical necessity. Two formats are commonly used:

A. Supplemental insurance forms are commercially available from health-care supply firms. These are preprinted forms with questions and spaces to provide the appropriate answers.

B. Individually drafted reports should include subjective findings, history and complications, initial examination, initial impression, and treatment plan. They should be brief reports, not narratives.

Interim Reports

Interim reports may be requested by the patient, insurance companies, or attorneys during the course of patient care. This kind of report is used only if an initial report has already been done. It serves to update the requesting party on the progress and status of the patient. Detail already provided in the initial report need not be repeated. Document whether the care is progressing according to the plan. Note if an update exam has been done, showing any positive findings. Note impressions and prognoses at the time of the report. Has it changed any since the initial report? State the current plan of care.

Narratives

A narrative is a detailed report developed in an orderly descriptive format. There are three styles of narrative forms. A narrative differs from an initial report in that it is an in-depth study of a patient's history of care as opposed to an overview. A narrative also includes a prognosis. When preparing the prognosis use specific language, for example, "guarded," "shows improvement," "possibility." Commitments to "guarantees" of cure are to be avoided.

Outline Narrative Form

The first type of narrative form is the outline form. An example of an outline narrative form would be:

A History/Complications
    1. Accident history
    2. Past medical history
    3. Was patient treated elsewhere at time of accident?
B. Subjective findings
    1. Symptoms as described by patient
    2. Are symptoms aggravated in any way?
C. Objective findings
    1. Physical appearance of patient (for example, include gait, any physical restrictions due to the accident, genetic handicaps, bruising, or lacerations)
    2. Postural evaluation
    3. Range-of-motion studies
    4. Neurological signs & tests
    5. Orthopedic signs & tests
    6. Palpation findings
    7. X-ray studies (includes subluxations)
    8. Labs
D. Original diagnosis (with ICD-9 codes)
E. Current diagnosis, if different (with ICD-9 codes)
F. Treatment plan/progress
G. Restrictions of activity
H. Basis of opinion
    1. History of injury
    2. Clinical findings
    3. Patient's complaints
    4. Review of medical history
    5. Patient's response to treatment to date
I.   Comments (For example: "It is my opinion, based on the accident history presented, patient history, and examination findings, that the patient's condition is a direct result of the injury incurred on [date of accident].")
J.   Prognosis

Fill-in Narrative Form

Fill-in-the-blank narrative forms are available on the market. When co-operating with, and relying on, an assistant to develop the text of the narrative, this approach may be an appropriate option. The doctor fills in the blanks and the assistant drafts the statements into text form. The format is somewhat restrictive, however, and may make editing in special situations more difficult. As with the other formats, after the final draft of the report is prepared, make sure a copy is placed in the patient's file.

Computer Form

This type of report is developed from a software package that helps create an in-depth record of the patient's history and the course of care. A questionnaire is provided for the patient and the doctor to complete. The results are then entered into the computer and a first draft is generated. From this first draft the doctor edits according to the individual case findings. Many times doctors have specific phrases or terminology they prefer to use in descriptive writings such as narratives. The narrative may require two or more revisions. With the word-processing abilities of many software programs, editing is very convenient. The end result is a thorough narrative that evolves from personalized editing. This system may save both doctor and staff valuable time.

Educating patients in the concepts of health and wellness is a constant, continuous task for everyone in the chiropractic office. Environmental factors in today's life make the task difficult, but not impossible. Use of positive, supportive attitudes and statements will help get the job done. Use of negative attitudes and statements about the patient or other health-care providers will not build confidence and trust. Instead, they will steer the patient away. Use of calm, balanced, reasoned thoughts and approaches to situations in statements offer the most certain path to long-term mutual support and admiration society relationships with our patients. Welcome to the world of being a change agent.

18

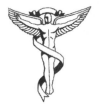 **Benefits for Owners and Employees**

Employee, or fringe, benefits are defined as any compensation other than wages or salary which is provided by the employer to the employee, the cost of which is tax deductible to the employer, and is not currently taxable income to the employee.

The topic of employee benefits is one of the most misunderstood subjects with which a starting entrepreneur has to deal. Often, even experienced business owners are not clear how benefit rules and the Internal Revenue Code can work to the advantage of the business owner. Many physicians want to provide benefits for themselves without incurring the expense of providing for employees as well.

Some benefits are forced on the entrepreneur by competitive factors in the personnel marketplace. Recruiting and retaining high-quality employees is becoming more difficult daily. Frequently, the competition showers the desirable employee with enormous benefit packages. Only meeting the competitive standard can keep these employees from moving to other opportunities.

Benefits are subject to nondiscrimination rules. The lawmakers' purpose in creating these rules is to insure that the business owner's fringe benefit is not out of proportion to the benefits for regular employees. The rules can be utilized to the advantage (read: higher compensation) of the owner, but may interfere with the owner's desire to be selective in giving benefits to some employees and not to others.

Because the subject matter is complex and involves taxes, a qualified adviser should be consulted. No entrepreneur can expect to stay up to date on the many rules and their frequent changes and still operate a health-care business. Staying current on tax and benefit laws, rules, and regulations is in itself a full time occupation. Therefore, most employers hire an advisor to assist them with plan design and implementation.

Broadly interpreted, fringe benefits include such things as vacation pay, coffee breaks and lunch hours, and free parking. This chapter assumes that the starting entrepreneur has already decided how to deal with those "standard" benefits.

Part-time employees may be excluded from fringe benefit programs. The definition of part-time employees, however, varies from benefit to benefit. Perhaps someday Uncle Sam and the various state governments will create a uniform definition, applicable to all fringe-benefit programs.

Group Life Insurance

Group life insurance is a frequently provided fringe benefit. Typically, it comes as part of the group health insurance program at the insistence of the insurance company, and the entrepreneur is given no choice but to buy it. Because the entrepreneur is the employee most likely to stay in the employ of the business, life insurance provided as a fringe benefit is attractive and can be integrated into the owner's personal life insurance package and financial and estate plans.

Under current law, premiums paid for the first $50,000 of group term life insurance on any employee are a reasonable, necessary business expense to the employer and are therefore deductible. However, they are not considered reportable (that is, taxable) income to the employee.

It is possible to provide more than $50,000 face amount of group term life insurance. The tax treatment is as follows: the premium paid is a tax-deductible expense to the employer; however, the portion of the premium for the excess insurance is reportable income to the employee. The benefit is still attractive to the employee, because the cost of the life insurance has been reduced compared to paying out-of-pocket premiums. The true cost is tax on the reportable income, or only a portion of the premium. The older the entrepreneur becomes, the higher the life insurance premium, the larger the difference between tax and premium.

Owner-employees may be provided with more death benefit than other employees, but there are limits. Current rules allow for two kinds of group insurance structures: a multiple of earnings for each employee; a classification by job category. An example will explain how this works:

Situation A (multiple of earnings): All employees are insured for, say, two times annual salary, rounded up to the next $1,000. Typically, the physician earns considerably more than the others, and thus is provided with a larger benefit.

Situation B (classification):

All corporate officers	$200,000
All non officer physicians	$100,000
All other salaried employees	$ 50,000
All hourly employees	$ 20,000

According to the nondiscrimination rules, if classification is used, no class may have more than 2.5 times the amount of the class immediately below it, nor can the top class have more than ten times the amount of the bottom class.

Group Major Medical Benefits Plans

Comprehensive group major medical plans are the normal health benefit provided by employers. After a relatively low calendar-year deductible, the plan will pay a portion (70 percent, 75 percent, or, most frequently, 80 percent) of the medical expenses incurred by the employee (and/or dependents) up to a certain limit of medical bills per year. Thereafter, the plan pays 100 percent of the expenses for the remainder of the years up to the policy limit.

The point at which the insurance company starts paying 100 percent of the bill is called the stop-loss or out-of-pocket limit. To illustrate, assume that the group major medical plan has an annual deductible of $250, after which the insurance company pays 80 percent of the next $5,000 of expenses. Then it pays 100 percent of expenses for the remainder of the year or until policy limits have been reached. The stop-loss figure, then, is $1,000, and the out-of-pocket limit is $1,250. Because of the stop-loss concept, the employee knows ahead of time his or her personal maximum cost on any medical bills during a given year.

The plans have family deductibles in addition to individual deductibles. These may be expressed as either a multiple of the individual deductible, or as a flat dollar amount that will be considered deductible for a family. The same approach applies to family stop-loss figures. They can either be a multiple of individual stop-loss amounts, or an overall amount, regardless of whether or not any individual's stop-loss has been met.

Nondiscrimination rules cause almost all group major medical plans to be written in such a way that all employees have the same benefits. Employers may require employees to contribute to the cost of the plan on a nondiscriminatory basis.

Since the late 1980s, various forms of managed care options have been included in the typical group health insurance plan available to the entrepreneur with a few employees. Originally, just the preferred provider organizations were included, today the point of services approach of HMO, PPO, and traditional major medical insurance is common.

Special Group Health Benefits

Major medical plans normally do not cover expenses for dental care, vision, or hearing care. In addition, there may be sublimits on such expenses as care for drug and alcohol abuse and mental and nervous condition care, as well as others.

Therefore, insurance companies offer separate group benefit plans for dental care, vision, and hearing care. These benefit plans require the employer to pay 100 percent of the premium for employees as well as dependents.

A common coverage is the prescription drug card. It is a "credit card" the employee takes to the drugstore to pay for the prescription. Only a small deductible (three, five, or seven dollars) is paid on the spot by the insured.

The appeal of the prescription drug card is that it pays for expenses which normally would not meet the major medical deductible. Most employees, at some time during a year, will purchase some prescription drugs. Typically, their cost, even if added to the doctor's visit, does not reach the deductible.

By slightly increasing the premiums for the group major medical plan, it is possible to provide for mental and nervous care, drug and alcohol abuse coverage, sterilization coverage, well-baby nursery care, and similar benefits. In some states these are mandatory coverages and are automatically included in the plan and premium.

When switching any of the group health insurance programs to a different insurance company, the employer must pay attention to the preexisting condition clause of the new policy. It is possible that, because of the switch, conditions covered under the old plan are not covered under the new plan.

Some group insurance plans limit or do not provide reimbursement for chiropractic care. We understand that chiropractors resent this approach. We find it nonsensical, however, for a chiropractor to insist that the benefit be part of group insurance they purchase for the practice, as they will then be paying premium for a benefit neither they nor their employees will ever use. Common operating procedure among professionals is to provide their professional service to their employees and families at no cost. It is considered a fringe benefit, much like airline employees can fly without paying for a ticket. No matter what percentage the plan would reimburse for chiropractic care, the reimbursement on a fee for service of $0.00 is still . . . ?

The Salary Reduction Plan

Officially known as the Section 125 Salary Reduction Plan, this benefit assists all employees. Sole proprietors or partners are not employees, and thus the owner can benefit from this plan only if the professional practice is a corporation.

The 1986 tax law changed the medical expense deduction for itemizing taxpayers, so that only expenses in excess of 7.5 percent of AGI can be deducted. Few taxpayers have that much in expenses, especially middle-class business owners in the health-care professions. The salary reduction plan allows the employee to take a reduced salary in return for which the employer agrees to pay for the employee's portion of the contributory health insurance premium and other nonreimbursed medical expenses. Limits on the reduction and reimbursement are imposed by the Internal Revenue Code.

Pension Plans

A variety of pension plans (more properly referred to as qualified retirement plans) exits today. All are subject to restrictions and limitations. This chapter will provide enough information on each type of plan to allow the entrepreneur to question the advisor as to the suitability and design of the plan. No tax or plan design advice is intended. Each decade, a number of changes occur in federal income tax law affecting pension plans. For that reason only (but there are others as well) pension plan administration is so complex that use of an advisor is a prerequisite.

Pension plans require the inclusion of full-time employees who meet minimum eligibility requirements. Any employee who has more than one year of service with the employer and is over the age of 21 is eligible to participate in the plan. "Ownership" of a participant's account is earned on a service basis. This is referred to as vesting. For each year of service (employment) with the employer a participant earns an increase in the vested portion of the account. The plans which health-care providers have are normally top-heavy plans. Therefore minimum contributions need to be made to the employee's account. Most entrepreneurs initially react negatively to this information. Upon reflecting, though, they realize that this nondiscrimination requirement can work in their own favor.

Any nonvested portion of an employee's account value will be distributed over the remaining participants' accounts upon termination of employment of the employee. Thus, in a practice with some employee turnover, the longer an employee participates in a plan, the larger the value of that employee's account as a result of redistributions. It is obvious that the employee most likely to remain permanently in the service of a business is the owner. Thus, the owner eventually ends up with the largest plan account. In reality, the nondiscrimination and vesting rules work together to build a larger account than could be accomplished without making contributions for the other employees.

An example will explain the concept. The vesting rules require the following schedule:

Years of Service	Vested Percentage
1	0
2	20
3	40
4	60
5	80
6	100

Assume that Sue Smiley has worked for Dr. Jones at the South Side Clinic for a little over three years. Further assume that Dr. Jones had to contribute $1,000 to the plan for Sue for each of the last two years (she was not eligible in her first year of service). Finally, assume there are no other employees participating in the plan. Sue's account value is now $2,250 including earnings. She will receive a vested benefit of $900, and the remaining $1,350 will become part of Dr. Jones' account. Without the contributions for Sue, the rules would not have allowed the doctor this extra "contribution" to his account.

It should be noted that Uncle Sam (and the state) assist Dr. Jones in making the contribution for Sue in the first place. Remember the definition of fringe benefits: contributions are deductible to the employer. If Dr. Jones' federal marginal tax rate is 28 percent, and his state tax marginal tax rate is 6 percent, then 34 percent of each year's contribution ($340) was paid for by the government. Thus, to pay Sue $900 in pension benefits cost Dr. Jones $220 ($900 minus two times $340) and increased his own account by $1,350. Not a bad situation.

Contributions to pension plans are deducted on the tax return from earned income prior to calculation of taxable income. Therefore the money is "saved" with before-tax dollars. When Uncle Sam allows this to happen, strings are always attached. The strings are: if money is withdrawn before retirement (which is defined by law as prior to age $59^1/_2$) the money will be considered taxable income to the individual and will be subject to a nondeductible excise tax of 10 percent of the amount withdrawn. This is called the early withdrawal penalty. Early withdrawal does not apply in case of disability (as defined by the Social Security Administration) or death of the individual receiving the early withdrawal. Upon retirement, moneys drawn out of the plans are subject only to normal income taxation.

All pension plans described in this chapter, except the IRA and the SEPP (defined below) are subject to annual reporting requirements. Each year the government and the participants must be informed of the status and changes in the plan. Most employers will pay their adviser a small fee for preparing the annual reports and returns.

Profit-sharing Plans

The profit-sharing plan is the most frequently used of the qualified plans. It allows an employer to determine the dollar amount of the contribution annually. Contributions are distributed to the participants' accounts in the same relationship as their compensation is to the total compensation of all participants. To continue with the above example, if Dr. Jones decides to contribute $6,000 each year to the plan, and if Sue earns one-fifth of the doctor's salary, then the contribution will be split $5,000 ($6,000 divided by 120 percent) for Dr. Jones and $1,000 for Sue.

The profit-sharing contribution is subject to maximums. An employer may contribute (and deduct on the tax return) 15 percent of each employee's compensation, but a contribution may not be more than $30,000 (adjusted annually for inflation) for any employee. Moral of the story: A profit-sharing plan can be a nice deduction on the income tax return. Keep in mind that the government will pay approximately one-third of the contribution by reducing the income taxes.

The 401(k) Plan

A special form of the profit-sharing plan is the cash or deferred compensation plan, commonly referred to as the 401(k) plan. Theoretically, the participant has a choice of taking the profit distribution in cash, which is not the intent of the employer. Therefore, the employer offers to "match," all or in part, any "bonus" the employee chooses to defer and contribute to the 401(k) plan. For example, if Dr. Jones offers Sue a $600 bonus at the end of the year, and promises to match it two-thirds ($400) if she defers it, he would make the $1,000 contribution to the plan. If Sue takes the bonus in cash, she would receive only the $600. Of course this $600 cash bonus payment is taxable income to Sue, thus she would receive only somewhere around $360 to $450 in cash (or check) after the withholdings.

The 401(k) plan may be of interest to the entrepreneur who feels that cash flow does not allow for profit sharing, but desires to make some form of retirement plan available to the employees. It allows for voluntary salary reduction, where the employee directs the employer to pay part of compensation to the plan instead of the employee. Thus, an employer can make a retirement plan available without having to contribute for the employees. The cost of plan administration (normally only a few hundred dollars for small plans) is the only expense to the employer. To avoid abuse of this approach, the law imposes restrictive limits on the amount of salary reduction which may be elected by employees, especially highly compensated employees, for example the owner.

Money Purchase Plan

The money purchase pension plan differs from the profit-sharing plan in only two respects. First, the amount of the annual contribution is determined by the plan. In other words, the entrepreneur and the advisor select the contribution (typically in percentage form) when the plan is adopted. Second, the maximum contribution is 25 percent of covered compensation instead of the 15 percent that applies to the profit-sharing plan. The dollar limit on annual contributions for each employee remains at $30,000.

The Stacked Plan

Some employers, after a few years in business and with a stable, predictable cash flow, want to make more than the allowable profit-sharing contributions, but are not willing to cast it in stone as the money purchase plan requires. A compromise exists for them. Two plans can be adopted, one a money purchase plan with a required 10 percent annual contribution, the other a profit-sharing plan with the flexible 15 percent maximum contribution. In this manner the maximum contribution of 25 percent can be made when cash flow and profits allow, but in "bad" years only the required 10 percent contribution has to be made. Of course the cap of $30,000 still applies to each employee.

Defined Benefit Plan

The defined benefit plan does exactly what the name implies: each participant is told what to expect from the plan at retirement. This benefit statement is expressed in the form of dollars of monthly benefit, or in the form of a percentage of preretirement earnings. The trouble with the defined benefit plan is that the annual contribution cannot be known until it is to be made. An actuary needs to calculate the annual contribution. He will take the following factors into consideration: benefit promised, current participant account value, years until retirement for the participant, expected earnings on the invested account balance. Only then can the actuary determine the contribution required for each participant and as a result for all participants. This uncertainty about the annual contributions causes only those employers with long-established, stable cash flow to consider a defined plan. As with the defined contribution plans (profit-sharing, 401(k), and money purchase) the law limits the maximum contribution to the defined benefit plan. The limitation is expressed as a maximum benefit that can be promised.

If there is a large difference in age and income between the owner-employee and the other employee-participants, the defined benefit plan will cause most of the annual contribution to be for the principal's account. As a result, this plan is sometimes used as part of a buy-sell funding for a practice, when the current owner is advanced in age and the new owner is young. This works extremely well if the seller does not really require a cash payment, but would prefer a pension.

Keogh Act Plans

The Keogh Act plans (sometimes referred to as the self-employed retirement plans or the HR-10s) are the pension plans for proprietors and partners. All the rules described earlier about design, vesting, nondiscrimination, and contribution limits apply to the Keogh Act plans. The distinction between corporate plans and plans for proprietorships and partnerships no longer exists in the tax laws. In the past, self-employed retirement plans were more restrictive than corporate plans, but law changes in the early 1980s removed the distinctions.

SEPP

The Simplified Employee Pension Plan concept is to have a limited pension plan which will be exempt from the reporting requirements imposed on the plans discussed so far. A SEPP can be created by any employer in a very simple written document specifying the amount to be deposited annually at the end of the business' tax year. All employees who have at least three years of service and are over the age of twenty-one will be participants in the plan. The maximum annual contribution allowed for each employee is adjusted annually for inflation.

IRA

The Individual Retirement Account, or Individual Retirement Annuity, allows certain individuals with earned income a deductible contribution up to $2,000 per year. The earnings accumulate tax-free while left in the account. The full $2,000 can be deducted only if neither the taxpayer nor the spouse is an active participant in an employer-sponsored retirement plan. For active participants in employer plans, the full deduction may be taken only if adjusted gross income is $40,000 or less for a married couple, or $25,000 or less for single persons. The $2,000 deduction is phased out as income rises, and disappears completely at $50,000 and $35,000 respectively.

For the entrepreneur with a young but growing family, an IRA can be looked at as a tax-favored savings vehicle, rather than a retirement plan.

A rough rule of thumb is that an individual in the 28 percent or higher tax bracket will accumulate more money utilizing an IRA than can be saved on an after-tax basis. This rule assumes a time period of at least five years, and interest earnings equal in both cases. It considers payment of the excise penalty tax for early withdrawal and the ordinary income tax on the amount withdrawn. Thus some people utilize IRAs as a savings program intended to provide college funds for young children a few years down the road. Of course an owner-employee of a corporate practice or a proprietor could do the same thing, at higher annual contributions, with the corporate or HR-10 plan.

One of the most frequently overlooked fringe benefits is the "bonus" IRA. For the selected employee the entrepreneur creates an IRA with a check from the business. This is reported on the employee's W-2, but is immediately deducted on the employee's tax return. The employee incurs no extra taxes, but has a tax-sheltered savings plan. Care should be taken to review the deductibility of the employer's IRA contribution. The bonus IRA is one of the few approaches still allowing selectivity in fringe benefits.

TSA

The Tax Sheltered Annuity, also called the Tax Deferred Annuity (TDA) or Tax Deferred Investment Plan (TDIP), is available to employees of educational institutions and nonprofit organizations. It is mentioned here only because many physicians are on college faculties or their spouses work for an eligible institution. With the reduction in 1986 of the availability of IRAs, the TSA has become more important as a tax shelter to such individuals. A complex formula determines the maximum each employee may contribute through salary reduction each year.

Other Possibilities

The above is only a partial listing of the possible fringe benefits available to the owner of a business. Insurance and investment salespeople are certain to approach the entrepreneur on such topics as the split-dollar plan, the nonqualified pension plan, or the reverse-funding plan. In addition, considerations for funding buy-sell agreements will surface at some time during the period of practice ownership. Though we made an effort to explain some concepts of employee benefits above, we have purposely stuck to the basic concepts. Providing more detail would only copy the efforts of others, some more qualified to enter the required technical discussion.

We have a concern, developed from years of observation of practice owners' lives. Almost daily the entrepreneur is approached by excellent, highly professional and capable salespeople. These fine folks offer to sell all sorts of investment and tax-advantaged vehicles. Too often, at least for our taste, the sales effort takes precedence over proper qualification of the prospect being approached. This is almost guaranteed to be the case if the business owner is somewhat standoffish and lets it be known that a practice management, accountant, or business advisor may need to be consulted on any such topic. Sales pressure suddenly mounts. We feel strongly that the security of a business can be damaged by committing too early or too heavily to any one investment approach. Our purpose in including this chapter is to provide the entrepreneur with some basics and some terminology, so that in these situations the practitioner can be strong. Realize this is a highly technical, complex part of business life. It is imperative that decisions are made wisely, slowly, and after much consideration of the available options.

Epilogue

The days are gone when the only requirement for starting a business was to hang out a shingle. Detailed study, planning, and determined implementation will lead to success. This involves a great deal of work, dedication, and fortitude.

Decide the structure for your business and design your critical path. You are not a specialist in every area of business, so enlist the professional services in your areas of need, for example, an accountant or an attorney, a business owner, or a clinician. You need to develop the mindset of an entrepreneur and address realities. Be aware of the legal requirements and of taxes, the necessity of having goals and objectives, and the importance of evaluating progress.

Clarify your practice philosophy. Develop your practice around that philosophy, do not stray from it, and progress steadily toward it. The image presented by you and your staff will promote that philosophy.

Develop a well-organized and structured business. Each of its parts—reception, accounting, insurance, and clinic functions—should work in harmony with each other. If the sparks of trouble that arise in day-to-day details are taken care of, many stress-induced forest fires will not develop. Internal and external marketing as well as public relations will lose their impact if your practice is preoccupied with survival. You must continually grow as a businessperson whose business happens to be chiropractic. Stay abreast of business developments within and surrounding your practice community. Be aware and knowledgeable not only of tax laws and changes, but of the issues elected officials are supporting or avoiding.

Be a leader in your practice and a contributing member of the community. Involvement is a key tool in business development.

Many traditional schools of thought have been presented in this text. Through experience, education, and open-mindedness the authors have tried to offer guidelines to enable the entrepreneur to make sound business decisions. Such decisions develop a firm foundation for your practice, and will, with less stress and more enjoyment, allow your practice to grow. We wish you good luck, a joyful life, and the inner strength to attain your goals.

Introduction to Appendices A, B, and C

Decision-making is a process requiring information. Proper data collection and correct interpretation of the information developed, therefore, becomes a management task. Managing with statistics developed in one's own practice is the best way to assure proper decision-making. Comparing a practice's statistics with those of the industry is helpful in developing a sense of the differences that result from personal preferences, styles, and priorities. Chiropractic industry statistics are hard to develop because most practices are "closely held," therefore, information is not in the public domain. While sources such as *Robert Morris* and *Standard and Poor's* provide some basic operating statistics, neither provide information which is very useful for the practitioner as those two statistic-gathering organizations publish information directed toward bankers and investors. In order to assist the beginning practice owner, three sets of statistics are being presented in the following appendices.

In Appendix A we present historical information about a successful practice in the St. Louis area. The doctor had graduated from Logan College in August of 1985 and had been an associate, or employee, of a chiropractor for two years. He felt he needed "seasoning" of his clinical skills before starting his own practice. In the summer of 1987 this clinician felt ready and began planning to start a practice and looking for an appropriate location.

The practice opened its door with one office on December 27, 1987. Construction of the space was nearly complete and treatment tables and physical therapy equipment had been delivered. The x-ray equipment, however, was purposely delayed until the beginning days of 1988. Thus, advantage was taken of an artificial tax timeline to be able to quickly expense some capital acquisitions using Internal Revenue Code section 179 expensing on both sides of the deadline of December 31. As can be seen from the first graph, the practice developed very nicely over the next few years. On January 2, 1993, the doctor opened a second office in another part of town specifically for PI patients. This office was—and is— not really his, he is an independent contractor paying the owner on a per-patient visit basis in lieu of rent (at this writing the agreement specifies $10 per office visit with a monthly minimum of $1,250. In addition, he pays double the actual cost of the film for each x-ray he takes using the facility's equipment). In this manner he really has two offices, each open three days per week.

Appendices B and C provide the same information for new practices. While it is pleasant to know what the operation of an established practice may look like, it is as important to realize that time and experience have an effect on operations results. It is unrealistic for a practitioner to expect the same results at the beginning of a career as may be expected after five or more years. Appendix B (Startup Practice I) provides the history of a new practice which clearly is developing the success patterns we all like to see. It opened its doors on August 14, 1994, after the doctor had graduated from Logan in April. He had taken a head start on the process by beginning the planning phase during his trimester 10, in early February 1994. Appendix C (Startup Practice II) shows that not all graduates immediately have the skills and attitudes needed to open a practice from scratch. The main difference between these two practices is that the doctor in B is constantly marketing himself by being involved in organizations in the community, while the owner of the practice in Appendix C expects patients to find his office without any work on his part. Will this last practice survive? Yes . . . No . . . Maybe. If the doctor continues with the current recognition (resulting in action starting about February 1996) that he *must* learn to be effective in at least patient relations (developing referrals from the few patients he has) there is hope.

As the reader has discovered, professional practices are characterized by high fixed-cost and low variable-cost (per patient visit) factors. Therefore, office visit counts become important. The process of making a living wage in practice is really rather simple: In order to take some money home there needs to be profit from the practice. Profit results from collecting more for services performed then is necessary to pay the expenses of the practice. Collections result from charging for services rendered, services can only be provided to patients during, an office or home visit. In order to have patients show up for treatment they must have been new patients at some time in the past. Thus, in our opinion the new patient statistic is the one that starts the process. This is not to diminish the value of the office visit count or the average patient visit statistic. We just want to indicate that without new patients no practice can survive and prosper.

A number of practice management firms rely on the calculation of a patient average visit to determine the patient relations effectiveness of a practice. In turn this average is supposed to prescribe changes in approach the doctor or the staff needs to make in encouraging patients to return for followup care and to accept the concept of wellness care (maintenance care, in the parlance of some). The authors understand and agree that preventative care of the human body is important to the bodily, mental, and emotional well-being of humans. They also agree that the concept needs to be sold to the average chiropractic patient, especially those entering care in the acute phase. They feel, however, that excessive reliance on a particular statistic of dubious value is not the way to achieve the desired attitude. To be open, in discussing the concept and usage of the statistic with a number of the principals in management firms, a different interpretation appears than in discussing it with practitioners who are "members" of those firms. The average is calculated by dividing the number of office visits of all patients for a specified period by the number of new patients during that time. A target average is then provided to the practice. Underperformance in weekly or monthly results requires (in the practitioner's interpretation of the management firm's dictum) a "harder sell" to the patient.

We feel that the calculated average has dubious value if used in any way other than for trend analysis. Graphing the average patient visit (APV) will demonstrate rather clearly that the time period on which the calculation is based has a material effect on the result of the calculation. For instance, the one-month average is much more variable then the six- or seven-month average (can you imagine the swing in the weekly average?). The maturity of the practice also has an effect on the calculation result. A new practice will generate a lower value then a practice of two, five or ten years' experience and exposure to the customer. The morals: first, as in all statistical analysis, trends are more important than individual data points. Second, remember that averages are in and of themselves worthless information. Only when we recognize their descriptive limitations do they become useful. Third, avoid dogmatism or tunnel vision, use the information in conjunction with other available data.

We hope that the graphs which follow in the three appendices assist the starting entrepreneur to a get a "feel" for the nature of a chiropractic office. As the health-care market continues to change, with managed care and cash practices in the chiropractic profession becoming the norm rather then the exception, realization of the economic and financial factors of this practice will become more important. Having a feel for the relationships of the operating factors will then become a crucial factor in the potential success of starting practices.

Appendix A
Annotated Statistics From a Successful Practice

The statistics presented in this appendix describe the historial picture of a successful established practice. The doctor first worked as an associate in another practice to gain experience, then began his own practice. These financial pictures illustrate the successful progression of a developing practice.

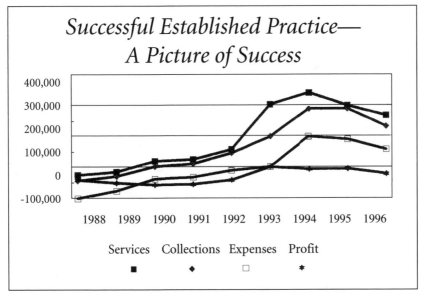

Fig. A.1. This graph displays nine years of the major practice statistics. A second office was opened on January 1, 1993 (3 days per week). Managed care effects seen after 1994.

Successful Established Practice— Selected Data

	1991	1992	1993	1994	1995	1996
Services	123,928	156,363	303,346	340,670	299,300	266,578
Collections	109,589	144,750	198,483	288,623	288,859	231,251
Expenses	43,131	56,644	98,908	91,250	92,618	78,869
Profit	66,458	88,106	99,575	197,500	188,550	155,382

Fig. A.2. This is the same information shown in Fig. A.1 in tabular form. Expenses have been well controlled. The change in collection ratio after 1992 is due to the PI business in the second office.

Successful Established Practice— Revenue

Fees For Services	1992	1993	1994
Manipulations	62,427	100,969	95,839
Other Office Visits	4,564	16,104	15,757
PT fees	90,840	166,500	170,100
Lab fees	1,022	529	444
X-Ray fees	20,120	33,100	30,587
Sales	1,107	3,827	4,059
Exam fees	7,220	17,200	22,400
Gross fees	187,300	338,229	339,186
Fees forgiven	(30,937)	(34,886)	(37,607)
Net fees	$156,363	$303,343	$301,579

Fig. A.3. Reviewing only total services may not provide enough management information. This breakdown of services will help in tracking what produces revenue. Other office visits include charges for paperwork (narratives, reports, etc.). Fees forgiven is the sum of the monthly accounts receivable write-off.

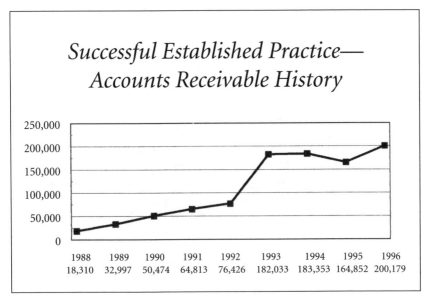

Fig. A.4. Accounts receivable rises with an increase in services. After opening the PI office, the jump indicates the time delay that is a natural part of that business segment.

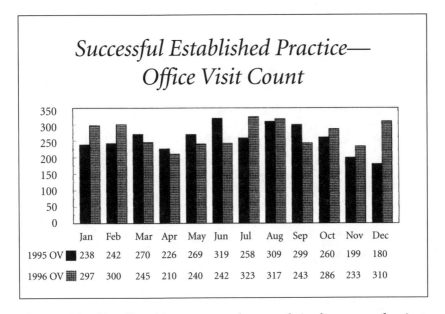

Fig. A.5. Monthly office visit counts can show trends in the success of patient education programs. Together with the new patient statistics they may be used for a number of derived ratios.

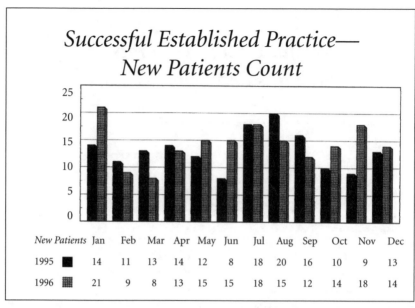

Fig. A.6. The new patient statistics show the result of marketing efforts. Together with the other stats, they can be turned into other evaluation tools such as patient visit average (treatment compliance) and average collection per new patient.

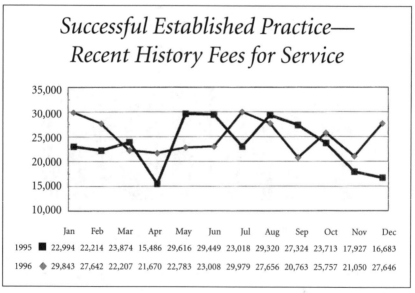

Fig. A.7. Tracking fees for service statistics can, when combined with the other stats, provide management information such as average visit charge, and average case value.

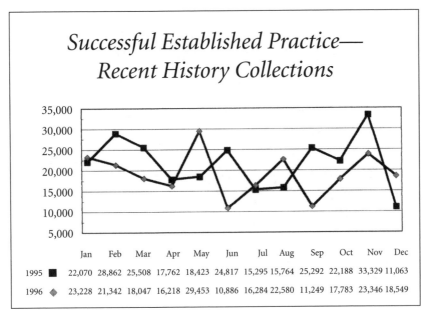

Fig. A.8. Collection tracking is crucial as part of cash flow management. In addition, average collections per visit, collection ratio, and others may be calculated.

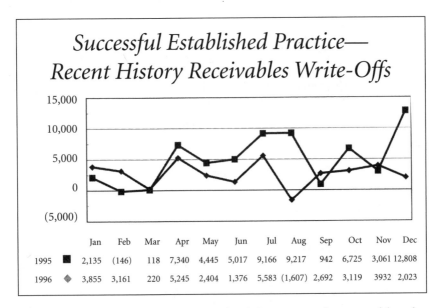

Fig. A.9. All professionals do pro bono work. It is important to be aware of the value of such efforts in order to judge the need for it in an individual case correctly. Patients do not appreciate the value of services for which they are not charged.

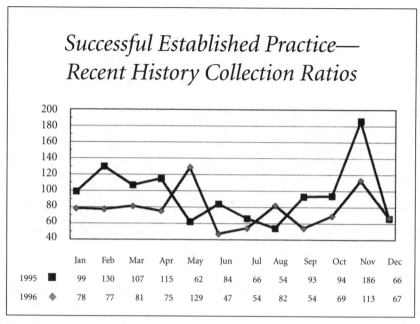

Fig. A.10. In a health care practice this ratio should range between 90 and 95%. In a PI practice it is difficult to get it above 85%. In a managed care practice 75% and above is good.

Managing with statistics will generate the information needed to make sound business decisions. It will develop a feel for the values and relationships of the practice. This sample practice has been well managed from a cost control point of view, successful marketing efforts and effective patient education.

Appendix B
Annotated Statistics from a Startup Practice With Success Patterns

Startup Practice I used in this appendix provides the history of a new practice which is developing success patterns. He began the planning phase while still in school. From the beginning he incorporated a strong promotional effort to increase patient volume.

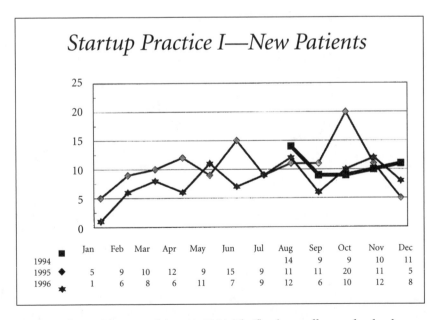

Startup Practice I—New Patients

	Jan	Feb	Mar	Apr	May	Jun	Jul	Aug	Sep	Oct	Nov	Dec
1994 ■								14	9	9	10	11
1995 ◆	5	9	10	12	9	15	9	11	11	20	11	5
1996 ✳	1	6	8	6	11	7	9	12	6	10	12	8

Fig. B.1. The practice opened Aug 14, 1994. The flood gate effect can be clearly seen. Family, friends, and patients who transferred from the school clinic create most of it.

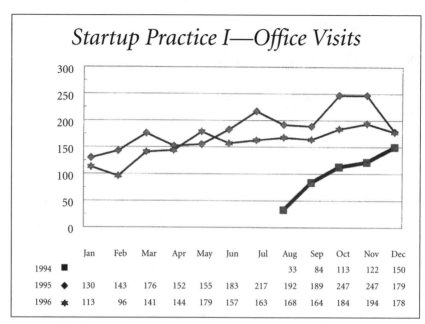

	Jan	Feb	Mar	Apr	May	Jun	Jul	Aug	Sep	Oct	Nov	Dec
1994 ■								33	84	113	122	150
1995 ◆	130	143	176	152	155	183	217	192	189	247	247	179
1996 ✹	113	96	141	144	179	157	163	168	164	184	194	178

Fig. B.2. Good patient education and adherance to treatment plan is clear. Average patient-visit calculations will not provide usable information in the first year.

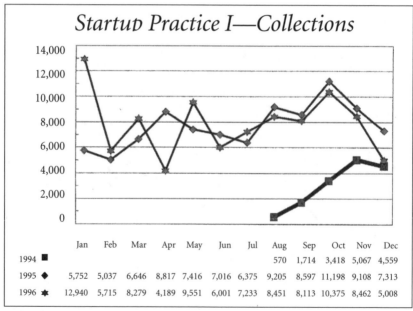

	Jan	Feb	Mar	Apr	May	Jun	Jul	Aug	Sep	Oct	Nov	Dec
1994 ■								570	1,714	3,418	5,067	4,559
1995 ◆	5,752	5,037	6,646	8,817	7,416	7,016	6,375	9,205	8,597	11,198	9,108	7,313
1996 ✹	12,940	5,715	8,279	4,189	9,551	6,001	7,233	8,451	8,113	10,375	8,462	5,008

Fig. B.3. A relatively high proportion of cash and health insurance patients helped this practice's cash flow early on. Deductibles and co-insurance portions are collected at the time of service. Don't be afraid to ask for it.

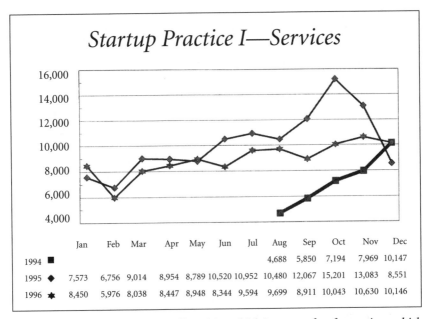

Fig. B.4. *New patients increase office visits, which increases fees for services, which increases collections, which allow the payment of bills and thus keep the doors open.*

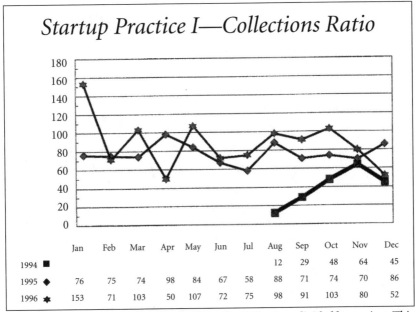

Fig. B.5. *This ratio is calculated by the formula: Collections divided by services. This ratio needs to approach 95% as soon as possible. The fastest way to raise the percentage is to ask for payment, preferably at time of service.*

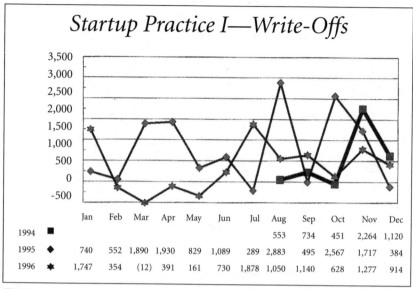

Startup Practice I—Write-Offs

	Jan	Feb	Mar	Apr	May	Jun	Jul	Aug	Sep	Oct	Nov	Dec
1994 ■								553	734	451	2,264	1,120
1995 ◆	740	552	1,890	1,930	829	1,089	289	2,883	495	2,567	1,717	384
1996 ✶	1,747	354	(12)	391	161	730	1,878	1,050	1,140	628	1,277	914

Fig. B.6. New practitioners too often doubt the value of their services and as a result will forgive fees too quickly. Therefore, keeping track of write-offs and fees that are forgiven is crucial information.

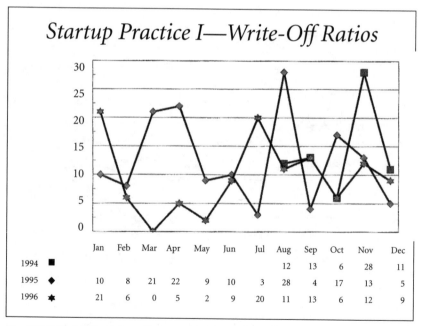

Startup Practice I—Write-Off Ratios

	Jan	Feb	Mar	Apr	May	Jun	Jul	Aug	Sep	Oct	Nov	Dec
1994 ■								12	13	6	28	11
1995 ◆	10	8	21	22	9	10	3	28	4	17	13	5
1996 ✶	21	6	0	5	2	9	20	11	13	6	12	9

Fig. B.7. Relating the write-offs to services more clearly shows the the starting physician the free services that are provided.

Appendix C
Annotated Statistics from a Startup Practice Without Success Patterns

Startup Practice II shows that not all graduates immediately have the skills needed to open a practice from scratch. The owner of this practice expects patients to find his office without any work on his part.

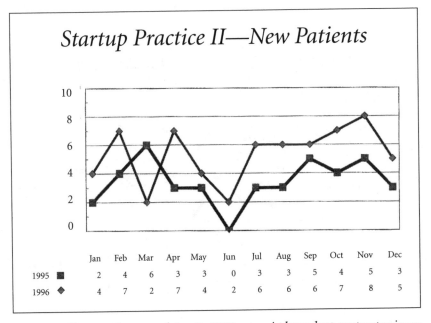

Fig. C. 1. The practice opened Jan 3, 1995 as an independent contractor in an established office. By May the doctor was dissatisfied with the situation and opened his own office in July.

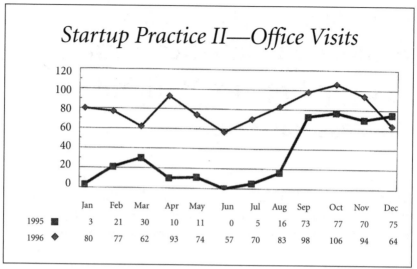

Fig. C. 2. A treatment plan that was too short and a patient noncompliance rate that was too high, hurt this practice in its early months.

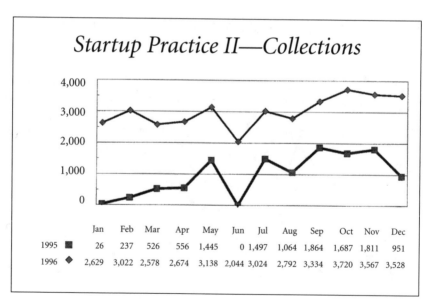

Fig. C. 3. The practice did not have enough patients, office visits, services, or collections. With expenses initially at $1,800 and then increased to $3,800 per month, this pattern spells trouble.

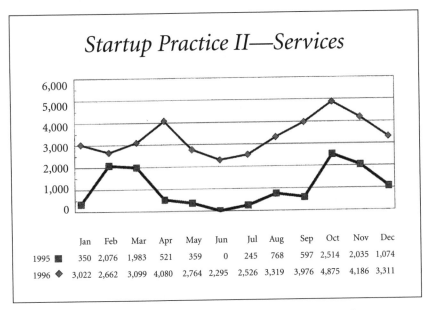

Fig. C. 4. Another sign of trouble. What needs to be done to improve?

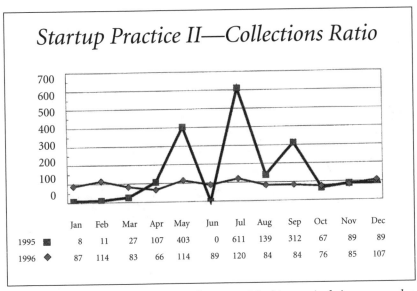

Fig. C. 5. Have you ever seen such a roller coaster? Is this practice being managed or is it just allowed to develop?

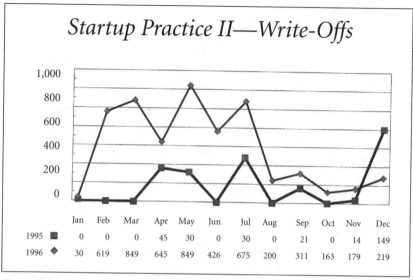

Fig. C. 6. *There are no services, and no write-offs. There is good and bad in everything.*

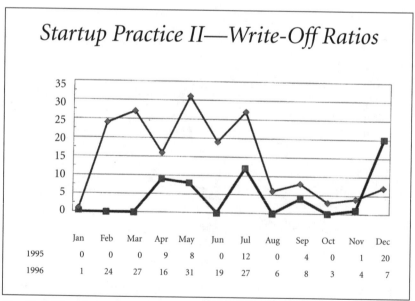

Fig. C. 7. *The picture remains the same in percentage format—no services, no write-offs.*

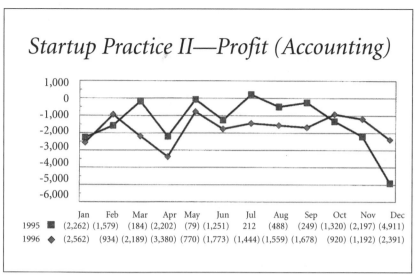

Fig. C. 8. Is this a livable wage? How long can this be sustained? How deep is the pocket?

The doctor owning this practice, an experienced corporate executive prior to entering chiropractic school, has an advantage over most new graduates. At his age and in his financial condition he can afford to wait it out. This pattern of practice development or growth occurs too often to individuals who do not have the capacity to survive it. As we have indicated throughout the text, marketing of the practice is crucial, especially in the beginning. Marketing requires that the doctor becomes involved in the community and meets potential patients. Professionals have never been able to hang out the shingle and wait.

If the patterns of this appendix show up in the early months of your practice, the best solution is to become an active marketer of your office and yourself. Use your skills and resources. Any discomfort with being out in public will disappear rather quickly. Escaping into expensive advertising programs will not produce the required results, it takes personal involvement in the community. If you doubt this advice, consult a practice management firm. They will confirm the suggestion, but at a much higher price.

Cautionary Note for Appendices D and E

Many students and practitioners ask for sample contracts and agreements. In order to provide some guidance to those not having been in a situation before, the authors have contacted friends and clients for the agreements used in actual practice. The following two independent contractor agreements are provided with some trepidation. Agreements and contracts should contain exactly what is agreed to between the parties. Our suggestion is to keep them simple and short. Trying to cover all possible future occurrences is an exercise in futility. Relationships between peers are continually changing. The authors feel it is good business practice to review the wording of agreements and contracts on a regular basis (say, annually) to assure that the paperwork keeps up with actual practice.

We are convinced that the initial draft of the agreement or contract needs to be written by the parties. This draft then needs to be reviewed and discussed, most likely amended, by the parties. Only when all parties are comfortable with the written document is it appropriate to visit a qualified business attorney for assistance. Attorneys, like most professionals, specialize. Thus be sure that the attorney has experience in the area of contract law. Most frequently one will find the requisite expertise in a business and tax attorney. Some real estate attorneys may be proficient in this area also. The attorney needs to be asked at least the following questions:

- Is it legal? After all, who wants to be party to an illegal contract/ agreement.
- What did we overlook? Attorneys see lots of business situations and dissolutions. Therefore they may be able to preview some of the pitfalls created by the document through omission or commission. It is perfectly all right for parties to an agreement to react to such an omission or commission with something like, "Yes, thank you, we thought about that but decided to do it this way/to not deal with that possibility."

- If this agreement leads to a lawsuit at some time in the future, will you take either side in the suit? This question tries to discover an imbalance or inequity in the agreement. Most attorneys want to take the side with the legal advantages.

The reader should note that the employment contract contains a Covenant Not to Compete, while the independent contractor agreement does not. The nature of independent contractorship is that we are already in competition, while the nature of the employment relationship is that one is boss and the other takes compensation for services rendered to the boss.

Final note: The agreements we present in the following appendices were not drafted by the authors, they come from the field. Neither author is an attorney, nor do we practice law without a license. Our sole purpose in providing these samples is to give the reader a feel for the appearance and content of agreements that work in the real world.

Appendix D
Ideal Employment Contract

Chiropractic Physician Employment Agreement

This agreement made this first day of January 1996, by and between Long Chiropractic Health Center, P.C., hereafter called the company, and John White, D.C., hereafter called chiropractor, state all the agreements, terms, and conditions between the parties.

Company is in the business of providing health care, specifically, chiropractic care, at its facilities located at 1234 James Street, St. Louis, Missouri, hereafter referred to as premises.

Company agrees to employ the services of chiropractor as an employee of the company and agrees to provide equipment, supplies, and paraprofessional staff as necessary for the purpose of providing chiropractic health care for the public of St. Louis.

Chiropractor accepts employment by company and agrees to perform professional services as defined by the laws of the State of Missouri and the ethical and professional standards of the profession.

Responsibilities

Company shall make space, equipment, and supplies and staff available for use by chiropractor on a nonexclusive basis. Company shall assign established patients of the practice to chiropractor and shall assign additional new patients on a fair, rotating basis with other chiropractors practicing on premises. All patients specifically referred to chiropractor by his assigned patients and generated by his personal marketing and promotional activities shall be assigned to chiropractor. Chiropractor agrees not to interfere with, or to disrupt or disturb, any pre-established doctor-patient relationships in company, nor any established business contacts, insurance-provider arrangements, promotions and other practice development programs of company or others employed by company. Chiropractor agrees not to be directly or indirectly employed by, or in any manner associated with, any other business or entity involved in health care (chiropractic or otherwise) without express written prior consent of company. Company shall not unreasonably withhold such consent, however, company will not consent to any form or relationship which it deems, in its sole discretion, to be of a competitive nature. Chiropractor is not authorized to, nor is responsible for, disciplining or terminating or hiring any company employee.

Advertising and Marketing

Company has provided and may, in its sole discretion, continue to provide certain advertising and marketing programs in support of its business operations. It is anticipated that chiropractor will provide additional marketing and promotional activities for company.

All marketing and promotional activities and materials require prior approval by company, even if chiropractor will bear the costs thereof. Chiropractor will make himself available beyond normal business operating hours for marketing and promotional activities initiated by company.

Accounting

Company shall provide chiropractor a monthly producer report detailing services performed, payments collected, and account adjustments made. Quarterly reports of accounts receivable, aging analysis, and other appropriate information relevant to chiropractor's employment and compensation may be provided at chiropractor's request. All accounts receivable are and shall remain the property of company, chiropractor has no rights with regards to these. Company shall have sole discretion in managing and collecting accounts receivable and in setting practice financial policies and fee schedules. Company shall have sole discretion in determining whether or not to employ collection agencies, which ones to employ, whether to institute any collection action, how or when to settle past due accounts, and any other financial or management decision making required in the operation of company.

Compensation

Chiropractor shall be compensated for his services rendered according to the following compensation schedule:

- Forty percent of the first $100,000 of annual revenues (in each calendar year) from chiropractic and related services rendered by chiropractor and collected by company;

- Plus, fifty percent of annual revenues (in each calendar year) between $100,000 and $200,000 generated from chiropractic and related services rendered by chiropractor and collected by company;

- Plus, fifty-five percent of annual revenues (in each calendar year) in excess of $200,000 generated from chiropractic and related services rendered by chiropractor and collected by company.

Compensation shall be paid on a monthly basis on or before the 10th of the month and shall be based on the collections of the prior calendar month. Compensation shall continue following termination of this contract on the above schedule for as long as collections for services rendered by chiropractor continue. Chiropractor shall have the right to review the accounting records, including patient ledgers, upon request. Chiropractor agrees to cooperate fully in all endeavors by corporation to collect fees for services rendered.

In accordance with federal and state laws and regulations, company shall deduct from chiropractor's compensation all required withholding and company shall remit such withholdings in compliance with applicable regulations in a timely fashion. In addition, company shall pay all required other payroll related taxes to appropriate federal, state, and city taxing authorities. Company shall maintain, and pay required premiums for worker's compensation or employers liability insurance as required by state law of the State of Missouri.

Should company adopt any employee benefit programs at some time in the future, chiropractor will participate to the minimum requirements of the plan in order for company to qualify for group plan benefits or to qualify for appropriate tax treatment. Any contributions (premiums, deposits, and such) made or required to be made on behalf of chiropractor will be deducted from chiropractor's compensation.

Proprietary Information

It is understood by both parties that in the course of performing services pursuant to this contract, chiropractor may gain access to company's office, operating policies and procedures, patient lists, referral sources, patient files, insurance-provider arrangements, and other proprietary information. Chiropractor agrees not to disclose, release, copy, or distribute, both during and after the period covered by this contract, such information or data for chiropractor's personal gain, other than necessary for performing the duties and responsibilities of this contract.

Malpractice and Liability Insurance

Chiropractor agrees to provide company's malpractice/professional errors and omissions insurance carrier with all required information to assure proper coverage for chiropractor and company. Chiropractor will cooperate with any of company's insurance carrier representatives and/or attorneys in order to assure proper defense of both company and chiropractor at time of claim.

Covenant Not to Compete

Chiropractor covenants and agrees, for a period of two years from the date of termination of this contract, not to directly or indirectly maintain an office or otherwise render chiropractic or related health care services within a ten-mile radius of premises, or future additional premises, of company. Chiropractor further agrees not to alienate any patient or to disturb any doctor-patient relationship of anyone associated with company during said period. Chiropractor recognizes and acknowledges that the business and affairs of the company, its patients and its methods of operations, are valuable and confidential and that unauthorized use or disclosure thereof, or violation of this covenant not to compete, would irreparably damage company. Accordingly the parties agree that in the event chiropractor breaches or violates any provision of this covenant, company shall be, in addition and as supplement to any and all other rights and remedies, entitled to an order or degree of specific performance of this covenant. Company may also obtain any injunction, enjoining and restraining chiropractor from the continuation of any act prohibited herein, to be issued by any court of law or equity having jurisdiction. The parties agree that company's remedies for breach of this covenant by chiropractor shall be cumulative and that the seeking or obtaining of injunctive relief shall not preclude a claim or award for damages or other relief. In the event of the breach of any provision of the covenant by chiropractor, company shall be entitled to recover all reasonable expenses, including attorney's fees and costs incurred by it in seeking to enforce the covenant or related actions.

No waiver of any breach of any portion of this covenant shall be deemed a waiver of any subsequent breach, nor shall it in any way limit the rights of either party to enforce this covenant. This covenant shall not be construed as an employment contract for any particular term and it is expressly understood that both chiropractor and company are free to terminate the employment relationship as determined in the appropriate section of the agreement. If any provision of this covenant shall, for any reason, be held to be invalid or unenforceable, such invalidity shall be confined to the provision hereof directly involved.

Termination of the Agreement

Company and/or chiropractor may terminate this agreement by giving thirty (30) days' written notice to the other at the last known mailing address or by giving personal delivery. The company retains the right to terminate this notice without prior notification in case chiropractor engages in unprofessional or unethical behavior, provides substandard chiropractic care as normally defined in the profession, or fails to maintain proper license to render chiropractic and related services. Upon termination of the agreement all patient files and related information and documentation will remain the property of company and chiropractor agrees to immediately transfer to company all such files, x-rays, patient lists, addresses and phone numbers and any and all other information or documentation in his or her procession.

General

This agreement shall be construed and the validity, performance, and enforcement hereof shall be governed by, the laws of the State of Missouri. This agreement may be changed, modified, rescinded or amended in writing attached hereto and signed by both parties. Should any provision of this agreement be held or declared invalid or illegal, the validity of the remaining parts, terms, or provisions shall not be affected. The waiver, by either party, of any part or the breach of any part or provision of this agreement shall in no way operate to, or be construed as, a waiver of any subsequent or other part or provision of this agreement.

Signed, this 24th day of November, 1996, at St. Louis, Missouri,

_____   _____

John White, D.C.   James Smith, D.C.
                                           President, Long Chiropractic
                                           Health Center, P.C.

Appendix E
Sample Ideal Independent Contractor Agreements

Sample Agreement One

Independent Contractor Agreement

I. Principals and Place of Business

The principals and parties involved are as follows: Dr. George Young, D.C., sole proprietor of Young Chiropractic, whose place of business is 2107 Jamestown Road, in the county of St. Louis, Missouri. Hereafter Dr. George Young, D.C., shall be referred in this document as Lessor. Dr. Henry Albright, D.C., independent contractor residing at 112 Front street, Apt 1, St. Louis, Missouri, in the county of St. Louis. Hereafter, Dr. Henry Albright, D.C., shall be referred to as Lessee.

The place of business shall be Young Chiropractic, located at 2107 Jamestown Road in the county of St. Louis. Hereafter the place of business shall be referred to as Young Chiropractic. Young Chiropractic shall be used to signify the location of the practice, only. In this document, Young Chiropractic does not refer to any assets, liabilities, or equity, (including but not limited to equipment and patient files), which are property of Lessor under Young Chiropractic, the entity.

II. Definitions, Legalities, and Miscellaneous

This is a legal and binding agreement by and between Lessor and Lessee. Any alterations, changes, or additions to this document are not binding unless these procedures are followed: Any alterations, deletions, or additions made must be made and initialized by Lessor, Lessee, and one witness. In addition, section XI must be completed and signed by lessor, lessee, and a witness. A photocopy of this document is not valid. This agreement shall be signed in triplicate with three originals.

III. Term and Effective Date

The term of this agreement is one year. This agreement may be renewed annually using the addendum following the end of this agreement. The effective date of this agreement is September 1, 1996. Any usage of Young Chiropractic by Lessee prior to the effective date shall not be covered to this agreement.

Lessor and Lessee both have the right to terminate this contract at any time with forty-five (45) days' written notice. Lessor has the right to waive this notice with consent of Lessee. Lessee has the right to waive this notice with consent of Lessor.

IV. Usage and Occupancy

A. Lessee shall have use of Young Chiropractic for the purpose of practicing Chiropractic as described by the State of Missouri. In addition to usage of Young Chiropractic, Lessee shall have the right use to the following:

> Any and all equipment as of the occupancy date
>
> Office supplies (see office paperwork)
>
> Office paperwork—Much of the office paperwork has the Young Chiropractic logo. Lessee may use this paperwork. Any changes to this paperwork may be done, with permission of Lessor, at Lessee's expense.
>
> Patient supplies (except radiological film and other patient supplies above and beyond the existing supplies)
>
> Utilities
>
> Computer equipment
>
> Office marketing aids, literature, etc.
>
> Texts, literature, etc.

B. Lessee shall have the right to use Young Chiropractic at will, within reason. Lessee shall set and keep his own hours, schedule and maintain his own patients and files, and bill and collect his own fees. It is strongly encouraged that Lessee and Lessor agree on office hours prior to posting and changing.

C. This agreement does not include such items as (but not limited to): accounting fees, legal fees, insurance (liability and malpractice), or any other service fees or insurance fees.

V. Restrictions

The following restrictions apply to Lessee:

A. Lessee may not solicit business through patients or patient families and friends of Lessor or any other professional working at Young Chiropractic.

B. Lessee may not use collections received for Lessor or any other professional working at Young Chiropractic for personal gain. This is a violation of federal law.

C. Lessee may not make long-distance calls using Lessor's telephone lines for any purpose without consent of Lessor prior to each individual use. Payment for these usages shall be made by Lessee to Lessor as soon as Lessor bills Lessee.

D. Any alterations to the facility, design of the facility, or rearrangement of Young Chiropractic without consent of Lessor is prohibited. Such alterations, designs, or rearrangements that are approved by Lessor shall be done at Lessee's expense, unless otherwise agreed upon.

E. Any and all belongings of Lessee which are on the premises of Young Chiropractic are the responsibility of Lessee to police and maintain. Such belongings are there at Lessee's own risk, and Lessor is not responsible for damages or maintenance of these properties.

F. Any belongings of Lessee brought or kept at Young Chiropractic may be subject to usage by other professionals working at Young Chiropractic. If Lessee does not wish for other professionals to utilize these belongings Lessee must notify Lessor prior to bringing the belongings on the premises. Lessor has the right to approve or disapprove any belonging to be kept on these premises.

The following restrictions apply to Lessor:

A. Lessor may not solicit business through patients or patient families and friends of Lessee.

B. Lessor may not use collections received for Lessee. This is a violation of federal law.

C. Lessor may not make long-distance calls using Lessee's telephone lines for any purpose without consent of Lessee prior to each individual use. Payment for these usages shall be made by Lessor to Lessee as soon as Lessee bills Lessor.

D. Every effort shall be made by Lessor to make Lessee aware of any alterations made to Young Chiropractic. A maintenance fee may apply in addition to the standard rental agreement of Younster Chiropractic. These fees may not exceed ten percent (10%) yearly of Lessee's yearly payment amount.

VI. Costs

A. The fee for usage of Young Chiropractic by Lessee for the period September 1, 1996, through August 31, 1997, shall be $18,000.00. This shall be paid monthly at a rate of $1,500.00. This payment shall be due on the last day of the month for the first six months and due on the first day of the month for the last six months. Any moneys received five (5) days past the due date shall be deemed late and a late fee shall apply. This fee shall be one percent (1%) of the balance due per day from the due date. For example—Lessee has a $700.00 balance and is ten days past the due date, the additional fee shall be $70.00, for a total amount due of $770.00.

B. The usage fee does not include any additional fees described in this document. This usage fee does not include any business expenses incurred by Lessee. Lessor shall not be responsible for these expenses, nor shall he be liable.

C. Additional expenses shall be considered items such as: (But not limited to)
Radiological film—at $2.50 per film used
Additional therapy supplies not already used—at cost
Any orthotic, supplement, brace, or device belonging to Lessor—at cost
Any specific device, marketing aid, or product specifically bought by Lessor
and not intended for Lessee to utilize under standard arrangements—at cost.

VII. Responsibilities, Duties, Rules, and Ethics

Lessee shall be responsible to act professional while practicing at Young Chiropractic. Lessee is expected to be aware of and uphold all laws and ordinances which may apply. Lessee is expected to practice ethically as described by the Missouri State Board of Chiropractic Examiners. Violation of any of the aforementioned responsibilities are grounds for immediate termination of this agreement.

Lessee shall be responsible for his share of any necessary cleaning and organizing of Young Chiropractic. Lessee shall make every effort to maintain a friendly working environment conducive to health care and the operation of a business respected in the community.

Lessee shall be responsible for proper opening and closing procedures as those pertain to entering and leaving the place of business each day. Any gross failure to do so, which results in a significant increase in expenses to Lessor, are to be passed through and will increase Lessee's costs.

VIII. Common Office Management Procedures

A. Triage of New Patients—Any new patient who enters Young Chiropractic shall be considered a patient of Lessor unless otherwise stated below:

- A patient who is a direct referral to Lessee (direct marketing/contact solely by Lessee)
- A patient who is an indirect referral to Lessee ("a friend told me," etc.)
- A patient who has been determined to be classified as a walk-in at a time when it is known to be a time when Lessor does not have office hours. (As Lessee has a separate telephone line, patients who call in will call the appropriate number.)
- A patient referral from another professional at Young Chiropractic, due to technique, scope of practice, etc., as deemed by Lessor and Lessee
- Only in rare situations will a new patient not be scheduled with their assigned provider
- If it is deemed unavoidable for a physician to treat a new patient who should be a patient of a different physician, it is herewith allowed. This patient shall remain a patient of the original physician. Compensation to the treating doctor for such

services shall be fifty percent (50%) of collections for services provided that particular day.

B. Triage of Existing Patients:
- If at all possible an existing patient should be scheduled with their assigned provider
- The existing patient file, services of that patient, referrals from that patient, and collections from that patient shall be deemed the property of the assigned physician, regardless of who treats the patient on any given date of service.
- If it is deemed unavoidable for a physician to treat an existing patient who should be a patient of a different physician, it is herewith allowed. The patient shall remain a patient of the original physician. Compensation to the treating doctor for such services shall be fifty percent (50%) of collections for services provided that particular day.

IX. Disclaimer

All patient files are property of the assigned provider and are nontransferable without written consent of the patient. Written consent of the patient must also be obtained by any provider, including the assigned provider if that patient file is to be transferred to another facility outside of Young Chiropractic.

XI. Signatures

We the undersigned agree to the principal and terms of this agreement. We are aware that this is a fully legal document and will abide by its terms. We contest that this is the last and most current agreement between parties involved.

_____   _____
Henry Albright, D.C.   George Young, D.C.
Signature of Lessee   Signature of Lessor

_____   _____
Date   Date

Signed before my presence on this _____ day of _____ in the year 19 _____ .

Seal _____   My commission expires _____ .
     Signature of Notary Public

Addenda

A. Addendum 1

For the period of the first three months (September, October, November), in the event Lessee cannot make the full payment amount due, the remainder of the amount due shall become due with the next payment due date without penalty of interest. After the three-month moratorium is complete the remainder balance due shall become due in full with the next payment. Late fees and interest will apply starting with the December, 1996, due date, unless special arrangements are made, agreed upon, and initialized below by Lessor and Lessee.

This addendum is added and becomes effective on the initiation date of this agreement.

_____   _____

Initials Lessor   Initials Lessee

B. Addendum 2

C. Addendum 3

Facility Use Agreement

This agreement, made this 1st day of February, 1989, by and between South Side Clinic, a Missouri corporation in organization owned by Susan Choo, D.C., and Sherri Mayfair, D.C., and hereinafter referred to as "the practice," and Demetrius Davis, D.C., a proprietor, hereinafter referred to as "Davis," constitutes the entire agreement between the parties under which Davis may use the facilities and services of the practice to operate his (Davis') chiropractic business.

Davis agrees to rent from the practice the co-use of facilities and services during the following maximum weekly schedule:

Tuesdays	1:30 P.M. till 6:30 P.M
Thursdays	1:30 P.M. till 6:30 P.M.
Fridays	1:30 P.M. till 6:30 P.M.
Saturdays	10:30 A.M. till 2:30 P.M.

In addition, the facilities shall be available to Davis for emergency care at any time. Davis agrees to pay the practice the sum of $200 per week as compensation, payable in advance.

Davis will operate his proprietorship as he sees fit, without interfering in the operation of the practice. Davis will pay all operating expenses of his business, including but not limited to license fees, malpractice and other insurance premiums, marketing and advertising expenses, postage, long-distance telephone bills, beeper and/or paging service expenses, x-ray film and supplies, and any other expenses he deems necessary. Davis will be responsible for the recruitment of his own patients. Any patients calling or visiting South Side Clinic for the first time, and not specifically asking for treatment by Davis, shall be deemed patients of the practice.

The practice will assist Davis in operating his business, among other ways, by collecting fees from his patients. Any fees collected will be passed on, reduced by the rent and any other expenses owed, to Davis each Tuesday at 1:30 P.M., together with a complete accounting for the previous week. If, out of necessity or prior agreement, Davis treats a patient belonging to the practice or formerly belonging to Dr. Jeffrey Jones (the practice having purchased the rights to such patient files from Dr. Jones) Davis is entitled to receive 50% of the fees collected from such patients. The practice's 50% share of such patient fees will be in excess of the above-referred rent, as it represents file ownership value.

Davis will care for his patients in a professional manner in order to enhance the reputation of himself and the entire practice. Davis will assist in keeping the facilities neat, clean, and professional looking. Appropriate professional demeanor will be displayed at all times; dress will be what is expected of a physician in the St. Louis area.

The parties agree that this agreement shall have an initial term of six months from the date of this agreement. After the initial term, either party may terminate this agreement upon sixty days' written notice, delivered to the last known residence address of the other party, or to the business address. During such period of notice, both parties shall continue to honor all parts of this agreement. Should Davis violate this part of the agreement, he herewith agrees specifically to compensate the practice and pay any expenses the practice incurs for collection such compensation, including attorney fees.

It is further mutually agreed that, should either party wish to sell ownership in the business, the other party shall have right of first refusal. Such right may be exercised at the then agreed upon price. Should agreement on price not occur, the selling party may solicit offers from outsiders. Any outside offer must, however, be subject to this right of first refusal, at the same price and conditions as those offered by the outside party. Nothing in this agreement shall, however, be construed to infringe the right of the shareholders of the practice to buy-sell each other's shares, as called for in the buy-sell agreement of the corporation. Any such capital transaction shall be viewed, for the purposes of this agreement, as a no-change transaction, and the resulting entity shall be deemed to be a continuation of the practice hereunder.

Nothing in this agreement shall be construed as making one party an employee of the other party. Each party operates its own business, makes its own management decisions, determines its own practice hours (for Davis within the limits set forth above), and is responsible for its own accounting and taxes.

Both parties agree to hold each other harmless for any malpractice claims other than their own. Both parties agree to carry malpractice insurance with limits of at least $1 million/$3 million from National Chiropractic Mutual Insurance Company of Des Moines, Iowa. Davis shall request NCMIC to keep the practice informed of all transactions with regard to his policy. He shall deliver, within ten (10) days of this agreement, a copy of this letter to the insurer making such request. In addition, Davis shall name the practice as additional insured on his Business Owner's Policy which shall have limits of at least $1 million/$3 million for General Liability and which shall be issued by insurance company with an A.M. Best rating of at least A (Excellent) and a financial size rating of at least XIII. A binder or certificate shall be delivered to the practice within ten (10) days of this agreement. Failure by Davis to deliver either or both insurance documents shall cause this agreement to become null and void and Davis shall lose any rights hereunder.

Both parties, finally, agree that this agreement may be changed by mutual consent at any time. Any such changes shall be made in writing and shall be attached to this agreement.

Signed this 1st day of February, 1989, at Canada, Missouri.

For South Side Clinic

_____	_____
Demetrius Davis, D.C.	Susan Choo, D.C.
Proprietor	President

Appendix F
Valley of Death First Year Cash-Flow Projection

Explanation of Charts and Graph in Appendix F

On the following few pages we give an example of a detailed cash-flow projection for the first year of operations. It reflects an exercise in planning and budgeting which forces integration of a number of concepts which have so far been reviewed only separately.

Figure F.2 projects the cash inflows. In order to properly construct a cash-flow projection, one needs to know the expected results from the marketing activities, the treatment protocol, the fee schedule, and the financial policy proposed for the practice. In the example, we assumed the marketing results as indicated, an average eight-week treatment plan consisting of three visits the second week, two visits each the third, fourth, and fifth weeks, one visit each the sixth and seventh weeks, none the eighth, and a final, discharge visit the ninth week. While this is not necessarily the treatment plan we expect for a patient with an acute complaint when visiting a chiropractor, we have seen many professionals employ similar treatment plans. Using it has the advantage of conservative planning and forecasting: It may understate the average office visits per patient; it does not take into account any visits by wellness or maintenance care patients; both are likely to cause underprojection of actual cash inflows. The fee schedule employed is $125 for a new patient visit and $35 for a followup care visit. The financial policy assumes that 60 percent of the fees will be paid at time of service (cash practice, in the usual terminology) and the remainder, be it insurance assignment, third-party pay, or patient-budgeted payments, are received an average of eight weeks later. Major factors influencing the result of this projection are the number of new patients, the treatment plans, and the amounts collected for followup care visits.

Figure F.3 displays the outflows from operations. We have tried to estimate the expenses and the timing thereof. For example, rent is always due the first of the month, utilities most frequently around the tenth (sec-

261

ond week), telephone the twentieth (third week), and so forth. These two projections are next integrated on a third, entitled "Net Cash Flow" (Figure F.4). Two cumulative net-cash flow projections are developed: Cumulative cash flow from operations, to see how the patient-generated cash flow develops; and cumulative net cash flow, which includes such nonpatient factors as the business loan and the doctor's financial requirements. To give the reader (perhaps the banker) the correct impression, the doctor's needs are separated into living cash needs (draw) and the needs of paying for past debts (student loan payments). This separation is not intended to indicate that student loan payments are a business expense—far from it—but rather to explain that the draw is as low as is reasonable for the doctor/proprietor to survive. It needs to be noted that the cash flow from operations projections has turned positive (cumulatively) in the middle of the third quarter, while it will take the (total) net cash flow until the last week of the year to perform that feat. The graph in figure F.1 may make this easier to see than the tables.

In figure F.5 we provide an example of a loan amortization schedule. With today's spreadsheet programs those are created within minutes. Most programs include a template, thus it is only necessary to input the three basic factors: loan amount, interest rate, and length of the loan.

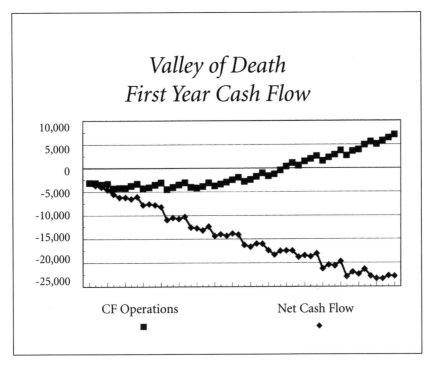

Fig. F.1. The net cash flow from operations and total net cash flow are graphed to display the working capital needs of the proposed practice. The values are sensitive to input factors such as new patients, treatment plan, fee schedule, financial polices, and operating expenses. Therefore, playing the "what if" game by creating multiple projections is a crucial exercise for developing an understanding of the relationship between business decisions and their effect on cash flow. If this graph is presented to outsiders, it might be best to rename it—Cash Flow Projection, for example.

First Year Cash-Flow Projection—Projected Cash Inflow from Operations
Purpose: To Discover the Valley of Death

Week	NewPts	OVs	NP$	OV$	TotalFees	Cash	ThirdParty	Deposit	CumDeposit
1	3	0	$375	$0	$375	$225	$0	$225	$225
2	2	9	$250	$315	$565	$339	$0	$339	$564
3	1	12	$125	$420	$545	$327	$0	$327	$891
4	2	13	$250	$455	$705	$423	$0	$423	$1,314
5	1	18	$125	$630	$755	$453	$0	$453	$1,767
6	1	16	$125	$560	$685	$411	$0	$411	$2,178
7	1	16	$125	$560	$685	$411	$0	$411	$2,589
8	2	14	$250	$490	$740	$444	$0	$444	$3,033
9	1	18	$125	$630	$755	$453	$0	$603	$3,636
10	0	16	$0	$560	$560	$336	$150	$562	$4,198
11	1	11	$125	$385	$510	$306	$226	$524	$4,722
12	2	13	$250	$455	$705	$423	$282	$705	$5,427
13	2	14	$250	$490	$740	$444	$302	$746	$6,173
TotalsQ1	19	170	$2,375	$5,950	$8,325	$4,995	$1,178	$6,173	
14	1	16	$125	$560	$685	$411	$274	$685	$6,858
15	1	15	$125	$525	$650	$390	$274	$664	$7,522
16	1	16	$125	$560	$685	$411	$296	$707	$8,229
17	2	15	$250	$525	$775	$465	$302	$767	$8,996
18	1	16	$125	$560	$685	$411	$224	$635	$9,631
19	2	15	$250	$525	$775	$465	$204	$669	$10,300
20	2	18	$250	$630	$880	$528	$282	$810	$11,110
21	1	20	$125	$700	$825	$495	$296	$791	$11,901
22	2	17	$250	$595	$845	$507	$274	$781	$12,682
23	3	20	$375	$700	$1,075	$645	$260	$905	$13,587
24	1	23	$125	$805	$930	$558	$274	$832	$14,419
25	2	21	$250	$735	$985	$591	$310	$901	$15,320
26	2	22	$250	$770	$1,020	$612	$274	$886	$16,206
Totals Q2	21	234	$2,625	$8,190	$10,815	$6,489	$3,544	$1,0033	

Fig.F.2. (first of two parts).

Week	NewPts	OVs	NP$	OV$	TotalFees	Cash	ThirdParty	Deposit	CumDeposit
27	2	23	$250	$805	$1055	$633	$310	$943	$17,149
28	1	23	$125	$805	$930	$558	$352	$910	$18,059
29	2	20	$250	$700	$950	$570	$330	$900	$18,959
30	1	21	$125	$735	$860	$516	$338	$854	$19,813
31	2	20	$250	$700	$950	$570	$430	$1,000	$20,813
32	2	19	$250	$665	$915	$549	$372	$921	$21,734
33	3	21	$375	$735	$1,110	$666	$394	$1,060	$22,794
34	1	24	$125	$840	$965	$579	$408	$987	$23,781
35	2	22	$250	$770	$1,020	$612	$422	$1,034	$24,815
36	2	22	$250	$770	$1,020	$612	$372	$984	$25,799
37	3	24	$375	$840	$1,215	$729	$380	$1,109	$26,908
38	2	25	$250	$875	$1,125	$675	$344	$1,019	$27,927
39	0	26	$0	$910	$910	$546	$380	$926	$28,853
Totals Q3	23	290	$2,875	$10,150	$13,025	$7,815	$4,832	$12,647	
40	2	19	$250	$665	$915	$549	$366	$915	$29,768
41	3	23	$375	$805	$1,180	$708	$444	$1,152	$30,920
42	2	23	$250	$805	$1,055	$633	$386	$1,019	$31,939
43	2	23	$250	$805	$1,055	$633	$408	$1,041	$32,980
44	2	24	$250	$840	$1,090	$654	$408	$1,062	$34,042
45	2	25	$250	$875	$1,125	$675	$486	$1,161	$35,203
46	2	25	$250	$875	$1,125	$675	$450	$1125	$36,328
47	3	23	$375	$805	$1,180	$708	$364	$1,072	$37,400
48	2	27	$250	$945	$1,195	$717	$366	$1,083	$38,483
49	3	27	$375	$945	$1,320	$792	$472	$1,264	$39,747
50	2	29	$250	$1,015	$1,265	$759	$422	$1,181	$40,928
51	3	28	$375	$980	$1,355	$813	$422	$1,235	$42,163
52	2	30	$250	$1,050	$1,300	$780	$436	$1,216	$43,379
Totals Q4	30	326	$3,750	$11,410	$15,160	$9,096	$5,430	$14,526	
Totals first year	93	1,020	$11,625	$35,700	$47,325	$28,395	$14,984	$43,379	

Fig. F.2. (second of two parts). This is one way to set up the revenue side of the cash flow projection.

First Year Cash-Flow Projection—Projected Cash Outflow From Operations
Purpose: To Discover the Valley of Death

Week	Rent	Utils	Phone	Postage	Wages	Prt	Ins	Supp	Repair	Adv&Promo	Prof Fees	Educ	Dues & Subs	Total Oper Out
1	$1,200			$64			$385	$800		$250	$300		$350	$3,349
2		$375												$375
3			$470					$125				$60		$655
4										$250				$250
5	$1,200						$35		$75		$125			$1,435
6		$150		$32				$55					$75	$312
7			$170							$250				$420
8														$0
9							$35				$125			$160
10	$1,200							$75		$250				$1,525
11		$200		$18					$50			$42	$12	$322
12			$170											$170
13							$35			$250				$285
Totals Q1	**$3,600**	**$725**	**$810**	**$114**	**$0**	**$0**	**$490**	**$1,055**	**$125**	**$1250**	**$550**	**$102**	**$437**	**$9258**
14	$1,200						$325	$175		$250	$125			$2,075
15		$200					$35							$235
16			$170	$32										$202
17										$250			$35	$285
18	$1,200				$110	$14		$150			$125			$1,599
19					$110						$125	$600		$835
20		$200	$170	$16	$110	$14								$510
21														$0
22	$1,200				$110	$14	$35		$80					$1,439
23		$200	$170				$35	$85					$35	$525
24						$14				$400				$414
25												$425		$425
26				$6	$110	$14				$200			$35	$365
Totals Q2	**$3,600**	**$600**	**$510**	**$54**	**$550**	**$72**	**$430**	**$410**	**$80**	**$1,100**	**$375**	**$1,025**	**$105**	**$8,910**

Fig.F.3 (first of two parts).

Week	Rent	Utils	Phone	Postage	Wages	Prt	Ins	Supp	Repair	Adv&Promo	Prof Fees	Educ	Dues & Subs	Total Oper Out
27	$1,200						$325	$150			$125			$1,800
28		$200			$110	$14				$200				$524
29			$170				$35						$35	$240
30					$110	$14								$124
31	$1200			$32			$150	$100			$125			$1,607
32		$200			$150	$20				$175				$544
33			$170			$35							$35	$240
34					$150	$20								$170
35								$175			$125			$300
36	$1,200				$150	$20				$175				$1,544
37	$200	$200											$35	$235
38			$170	$64	$150		$35		$50			$25		$489
39							$35	$100		$175				$300
Totals Q3	$3,600	$600	$510	$96	$820	$110	$430	$575	$150	$725	$375	$25	$105	$8,121
40	$1,200	$200			$150	$20	$325							$1,975
41								$155		$175	$125			$375
42			$170		$200	$26	$35						$35	$466
43									$125					$125
44	$1,200	$200		$32	$200	$26		$175		$400	$125			$2,158
45										$400				$200
46			$170		$200	$26	$35							$831
47													$35	$35
48					$200	$26		$225						$451
49	$1,200	$200		$12			$35			$175	$125	$225		$1,772
50			$170		$200	$26								$461
51							$450							$620
52					$200	$26		$150		$175				$551
Totals Q4	$3,600	$600	$510	$44	$1,350	$176	$880	$705	$125	$1,325	$375	$225	$105	$10,020
Totals 1st year	$14,400	$2,525	$2,340	$308	$2,720	$357	$2,230	$2,745	$480	$4,400	$1,675	$1,377	$752	$36,309

Fig. F.3. (second of two parts). Fig. F.3. Cash outflows are distributed to appropriate expense columns and correct timing is also indicated.

First Year Cash-Flow Projection—Projected Net Cash Flow

Purpose: To Discover the Valley of Death

Week	Deposit	Total Oper Out	NCF OP	CUMNCFOP	BusLoan	Dr.Draw	StdLoan	NC	FCumNCF
1	$225	$3349	($3,124)	($3,124)				($3,124)	($3,124)
2	$339	$375	($36)	($3,160)		$500		($536)	($3,660)
3	$327	$655	($328)	($3,488)				($328)	($3,988)
4	$423	$250	$173	($3,315)		$750		($577)	($4,565)
5	$453	$1,435	($982)	($4,297)				($982)	($5,547)
6	$411	$312	$99	($4,198)		$750		($651)	($6,198)
7	$411	$420	($9)	($4,207)				($9)	($6,207)
8	$444	$0	$444	($3,763)		$750		($306)	($6,513)
9	$603	$160	$443	($3,320)				$443	($6,070)
10	$562	$1,525	($963)	($4,283)		$750		($1,713)	($7,783)
11	$524	$322	$202	($4,081)				$202	($7,581)
12	$705	$170	$535	($3,546)		$750		($215)	($7,796)
13	$746	$285	$461	($3,085)	$875			($414)	($8,210)
Totals Q1	$6,173	$9,258	($3,085)		$875	$4,250	$0	($8,210)	
14	$685	$2,075	($1,390)	($4,475)	$582	$750		($2,722)	($10,932)
15	$664	$235	$429	($4,046)				$429	($10,503)
16	$707	$202	$505	($3,541)		$750		($245)	($10,748)
17	$767	$285	$482	($3,059)				$482	($10,266)
18	$635	$1,599	($964)	($4,023)	$582	$750		($2,296)	($12,562)
19	$669	$835	($166)	($4,189)				($166)	($12,728)
20	$810	$510	$300	($3,890)		$750		($450)	($13,179)
21	$791	$0	$791	($3,099)				$791	($12,388)
22	$781	$1,439	($658)	($3,757)	$582	$750		($1,990)	($14,378)
23	$905	$525	$380	($3,377)				$380	($13,998)
24	$832	$414	$418	($2,959)		$750		($332)	($14,330)
25	$901	$425	$476	($2,483)				$476	($13,854)
26	$886	$365	$521	($1,962)		$750		($229)	($14,084)
Totals Q2	$10,033	$8,910	$1,123		$1,746	$5,250	$0	($5,874)	

Fig. F.4. (first of two parts).

Week	Deposit	Total Oper Out	NCF OP	CUMNCFOP	BusLoan	Dr.Draw	StdLoan	NC	FCumNCF
27	$943	$1,803	($860)	($2822)	$582		$750	($2,192)	($16,276)
28	$910	$524	$386	($2437)		$750		($364)	($16,640)
29	$900	$240	$660	($1777)				$660	($15,980)
30	$854	$124	$730	($1047)		$750		($20)	($16,000)
31	$1,000	$1,607	($607)	($1654)			$750	($1,357)	($17,357)
32	$921	$544	$376	($1278)	$582	$750		($956)	($18,313)
33	$1,060	$240	$820	($458)				$820	($17,493)
34	$987	$170	$818	$360		$750		$68	($17,425)
35	$1,034	$300	$734	$1,094			$750	($16)	($17,441)
36	$984	$1,544	($560)	$533		$750		($1,310)	($18,752)
37	$1,109	$235	$874	$1,407	$582			$292	($18,460)
38	$1,019	$488	$530	$1,938		$750		($220)	($18,679)
39	$926	$300	$626	$2,564				$626	($18,053)
Totals Q3	$1,2647	$8,121	$4,526		$1746	$4500	$2250	($3,970)	
40	$915	$1,974	($1,060)	$1,504	$582	$750	$750	($3,142)	($21,195)
41	$1,152	$375	$777	$2,281				$777	($20,418)
42	$1,019	$466	$553	$2,834		$750		($197)	($20,615)
43	$1,041	$125	$916	$3,750				$916	($19,699)
44	$1,062	$2,158	($1096)	$2,654	$582	$750	$750	($3,178)	($22,877)
45	$1,161	$200	$961	$3,615				$961	($21,916)
46	$1,125	$831	$294	$3,909		$750		($456)	($22,372)
47	$1,072	$35	$1,037	$4,946				$1,037	($21,335)
48	$1,083	$451	$632	$5,578	$582	$750	$750	($1,450)	($22,785)
49	$1,264	$1,772	($508)	$5,070				($508)	($23,293)
50	$1,181	$461	$720	$5,790		$750		($30)	($23,323)
51	$1,235	$620	$615	$6,405				$615	($22,708)
52	$1,216	$551	$665	$7,070		$750		($85)	($22,793)
Totals Q4	$1,4526	$10,020	$4,506		$1,746	$5,250	$2,250	($4,740)	
Totals first year	$43,379	$36,309	$7070		$6,113	$19,250	$4,500	($22,793)	

Fig. F.4. (second of two parts). Fig. F.4. This is the final analysis sheet. The first two columns are copied from the prior spreadsheets. Net cash flow from operations and net cash flow are calculated. These are each accumulated to generate the graph on page 265.

Loan Amortization Schedule

Loan:	$25,000	Interest rate	14.0%
Monthly payment:	$581.71	Period:	60

Payment #	Interest	Principal	Balance
1	$291.67	$290.04	$24,709.96
2	$288.28	$293.42	$24,416.54
3	$284.86	$296.85	$24,119.69
4	$281.40	$300.31	$23,819.38
5	$277.89	$303.81	$23,515.57
6	$274.35	$307.36	$23,208.21
7	$270.76	$310.94	$22,897.27
8	$267.13	$314.57	$22,582.69
9	$263.46	$318.24	$22,264.45
10	$259.75	$321.95	$21,942.50
11	$256.00	$325.71	$21,616.79
12	$252.20	$329.51	$21,287.28
Totals 1st Year	$3,267.75	$3,712.72	
13	$248.35	$333.35	$20,953.92
14	$244.46	$337.24	$20,616.68
15	$240.53	$341.18	$20,275.50
16	$236.55	$345.16	$19,930.34
17	$232.52	$349.19	$19,581.16
18	$228.45	$353.26	$19,227.90
19	$224.33	$357.38	$18,870.52
20	$220.16	$361.55	$18,508.97
21	$215.94	$365.77	$18143.20
22	$211.67	$370.04	$17,773.16
23	$207.35	$374.35	$17,398.81
24	$202.99	$378.72	$17,020.09
Totals 2nd Year	$2,713.29	$4,267.19	
25	$198.57	$383.14	$16,636.95
26	$194.10	$387.61	$16,249.34
27	$189.58	$392.13	$15,857.21
28	$185.00	$396.71	$15,460.50
29	$180.37	$401.33	$15,059.17
30	$175.69	$406.02	$14,653.16
31	$170.95	$410.75	$14,242.40
32	$166.16	$415.54	$13,826.86
33	$161.31	$420.39	$13,406.46

Fig. F.5. This loan amortization sheet was used to generate the business loan payments in figure F.4.

Payment #	Interest	Principal	Balance
34	$156.41	$425.30	$12,981.17
35	$151.45	$430.26	$12,550.91
36	$146.43	$435.28	$12,115.63
Totals 3rd Year	$2,076.02	$4,904.46	
37	$141.35	$440.36	$11,675.27
38	$136.21	$445.49	$11,229.78
39	$131.01	$450.69	$10,779.08
40	$125.76	$455.95	$10,323.13
41	$120.44	$461.27	$9,861.86
42	$115.06	$466.65	$9,395.21
43	$109.61	$472.10	$8,923.12
44	$104.10	$477.60	$8,445.51
45	$98.53	$483.18	$7,962.34
46	$92.89	$488.81	$7,473.53
47	$87.19	$494.52	$6,979.01
48	$81.42	$500.28	$6,478.73
Totals 4th Year	$1,343.57	$5,636.90	
49	$75.59	506.12	$5,972.61
50	$69.68	512.03	$5,460.58
51	$63.71	518.00	$4,942.58
52	$57.66	524.04	$4,418.54
53	$51.55	530.16	$3,888.38
54	$45.36	536.34	$3,352.04
55	$39.11	542.60	$2,809.44
56	$32.78	548.93	$2,260.51
57	$26.37	555.33	$1,705.18
58	$19.89	561.81	$1,143.36
59	$13.34	$568.37	$575.00
60	$6.71	$575.00	($0.00)
Total 5th Year	$501.75	$6,478.73	

Fig.F.5. (continued).

Appendix G
Business Plan and Loan Proposal—Starting from Scratch

This appendix illustrates the form and components of a business plan and loan proposal for a startup practice. It includes the type of financial data that should accompany a business plan.

Player-Swanson Chiropractic

BUSINESS PLAN AND LOAN PROPOSAL

ALLYEAR CHIROPRACTIC

Quality Alternative Health Care Year Around

Business Plan: AllYear Chiropractic

Executive Summary
Marketing Plan
    Established Patients
    Personal Marketing
    Promotion
    Patient-oriented Management and Patient Relations
Principals and Advisors
    Bruce Player, D.C.
    James T. Swanson
    A. Fuller Jurist, Jr., J.D.
    Rudolf P. Vrugtman, M.B.A.
    John D. Smith, D.C.
Chiropractic's Position in Health Care
Business Format and Responsibilities of the Principals
Financial Forecasts
    Cash-flow Projections
    Pro Forma Balance Sheets
Milestones and Critical Factors
Financing Proposal

Business Plan
AllYear Chiropractic

Executive Summary

AllYear Chiropractic is the trade name for a Chiropractic Professional Corporation in organization. The incorporator is Dr. Bruce Player, who will have the charter application filed within days of receiving his license to practice in the state of Missouri. It is anticipated that AllYear will be open for the treatment of the first patients on June 15, 1994. The practice will be located in the AllYear Shopping Center at the intersection of Main Boulevard and Through Road, in West St. Louis County.

It is intended that the corporation, following the initial meeting, be owned by Dr. Player only for a period sufficient to allow Mr. James Swanson to graduate from Logan College of Chiropractic. Once Mr. Swanson is licensed to practice Chiropractic in the state of Missouri, and thus eligible to own shares in a professional corporation, 50 percent ownership shares will be issued to him per an existing agreement between the parties. This business plan has been prepared as if there are two principals from inception, as this is the attitude of the two individuals involved.

The startup process for any professional endeavor is characterized by two main factors. First, no matter how capable the professionals are from a clinical or business perspective, a period of negative cash flow exists in the beginning. Professional practices have high fixed costs relative to the variable costs per patient. Therefore, while the patient office visit count is low, cash flow will be negative. Second, the doctor-patient relationship is based on personal trust. This means that marketing strategies depending on advertising to draw threshold traffic may not be effective. This practice will rely on more appropriate marketing strategies that will develop long-term patient relationships. These strategies will, by their very nature, result in a slower initial growth in office visits, but should in the long run prove more profitable.

In this endeavor, cash flow and marketing will be the crucial factors in the first few years. The principals believe that they have, with the assistance of their advisors, developed plans and strategies to deal effectively with the pitfalls of starting a professional office. Using currently accepted financial measures, they expect to invest 38 percent equity at inception. The equity ratio will fall slightly during the startup phase to a low of 21 percent after a year and a half of operations, then quickly rebound to more than 60 percent after three years. Though opening day is still nearly two months away, initial marketing efforts have been started and will be the primary concern of principals and advisors for the next three years.

Financing will need to be arranged for the endeavor to be successful. Slightly over twenty-six thousand dollars will be sought in the form of a term loan for acquisition of equipment and initial supplies. In addition, a working capital line of credit of thirty thousand will be sought to assist in surviving the above described negative cash flow. At the time of writing this plan, two leasing companies have committed to provide the term financing.

Marketing Plan

Because of the nature of the relationship between doctor and patient, a relationship of personal trust which takes time to develop, the marketing strategies described below emphasize the two required factors: time and personal contact. While some kinds of advertising strategies will be employed, these will concentrate on name recognition and image development rather than the more immediate "action generating" style intended only to develop threshold traffic. In the experience of the advisors, patients drawn by threshold traffic advertising do not fit the target population characteristics of this practice, as they are primarily motivated by cut-rate fees and discount promotions, rather than quality health care provided with an eye on quality of life for the patient. Initial marketing efforts have already yielded a small number of "promised" patients at opening.

Established Patients

Five adult and two pediatric patients will follow Mr. Swanson from his current patient load at the Logan College Health Centers, where he is in his final internship phase of training. These patients receive manipulative treatment only, no physical therapy is normally performed on them. All pay cash at time of services. These patients will represent a total of seven office visits per week, generating approximately $350 in deposits per week. In addition, due to continuing discussions with others in his current patient load, an additional four or five adult patients can be expected to follow him to AllYear Chiropractic soon after opening day. These patients have a proven habit of referring others and will thus be expected to start referral as an immediate source of new patients. Dr. Player expects two adult patients to follow him to the practice from his internship period at the Yorkshire Clinic of Logan College.

Personal Marketing

Both principals are currently engaged in activities designed to develop local community awareness of the practice and the principals. Dr. Player has arranged to be guest speaker at a number of service organizations and frequently "visits" on a low-key basis with employers and business owners in the west county target market area. During these conversations he presents the recent Manga study results on the efficacy of chiropractic care in the worker's compensation area. He also discusses the well-established preventative care results provided by chiropractic care. Mr. Swanson will join in this marketing effort as soon as he has completed the very intensive portion of his internship responsibilities, which is expected to be completed around July 1, 1994.

Specific strategies to be employed:

Public speaking. The practice of speaking in front of groups and organizations increases visibility and recognition of the practice and its principals. It is almost required in today's health-care environment, besides, both principals are comfortable and effective in group communication situations. The costs involved in doing this are strictly time and energy. Preparation is required and might steal time from other marketing tools, however, no other approach has shown the positive results from a cost-benefit point of view.

Community involvement. Any business organization that receives support from its community is obligated to "return" the favor by supporting involvement of its employees. The principals intend to provide an example for future staff members by active involvement in selected organizations. While there certainly is a marketing angle to this involvement, selection of the organizations to become active in will be based primarily on personal preferences and philosophies. The costs are a time factor and relatively small membership and meeting dues. A list of possible involvement for the principals follows:
- R.C.G.A. and local Chamber of Commerce
- Managing children's sports teams (baseball—Dr. Player)
- Sponsoring and managing adult leagues (bowling—Mr. Swanson)
- Health club memberships
- Perhaps town/city council

Promotion

Advertising. This will include initial and annual open-house ads, wellness programs, image programs developing chiropractic and practice recognition in the community, and the like. Discounts and other fee reducing advertising, typically, is not cost-effective, as it draws the wrong kind of patient. Copies of advertisements may be mailed an average of four times per year to a select part of the target population with an appropriate cover letter. The outcome measurement of this particular marketing strategy is deceiving. While few new patients will be developed as a direct result of this route, existing patients may be encouraged to stay and may even feel comfortable referring others. The name recognition resulting from this effort should be invaluable in the long run.

Newsletters. A newsletter will not generate immediate new patient traffic. Instead, it is a strategy designed to develop image and name recognition and, if properly targeted, may cause "centers of influence" to refer patients. It may also maintain existing patients. To inform a target population of the status of the clinic and chiropractic is the primary objective. Patient education ultimately leads to referrals. Three quality newsletters a year will be the original goal. At five hundred mailed, the overall cost will be $930 yearly.

Allied Health Care Network. This network will be formed by AllYear Chiropractic. Its members would include interested doctors of various specialties, attorneys, and other related professionals. The main purpose is to provide a referral source to and from AllYear Chiropractic. The costs would include mailing, luncheons, and telephone fees, and should not exceed three hundred dollars per year.

Patient-Oriented Management and Patient Relations

Total Quality Management. This concept will be the theme of all activity of the practice. Quality is defined as responsiveness to the needs of the clientele. Regardless of how long a practice has been in existence, as long as it is continuously trying to improve, it will grow. Regular staff meetings will suggest operational and other factors requiring attention. Often, the patients will tell the staff members things they would never say to the doctor. Open and honest communication with employees will develop more ideas and suggestions than ever thought possible. In many chiropractic offices the progress of a patient is reevaluated after eight or ten visits. At AllYear Chiropractic, the practice will be evaluated by each patient, each time the patient is clinically reevaluated for care, thus creating two-way communication. Suggestions from these evaluations will be discussed at following staff meetings and, if appropriate, change in standard operating procedures or standard treatment protocol will be initiated. Costs are minimal (almost zero). Expected results would include a health-care office designed by patients.

Office Appearance. A professional appearance will suggest such thoughts as serious, successful, proud, compliance. To achieve this the staff must picture what the average patient perceives a friendly office to be. Cleanliness is a prerequisite. A dirty office does not denote health. Brightness is important, especially for people in pain and depression. Interesting wall decor might give an office a certain uniqueness. And clean, well-dressed staff is crucial for positive patient relations. Cleaning costs could vary, but might be estimated for five hours per week at six dollars per hour; yearly maintenance/decorations costs would be incurred in routine budget and lease arrangements.

Office Policies. Subtleties often represent the difference between a referral practice and a nonreferral practice; the details are that crucial. Many of these fall under the heading of general organization. Organization is expected in a professional practice and quality in organization becomes a marketing tool. Consideration for customers is likewise crucial. Showing patients that they are being considered is common sense, yet seldom done in the health-care industries. Some suggestions for AllYear Chiropractic include:

- Be sure doctors are available when a patient wants to talk to them (i.e., telephone, letters). Have a fail-safe plan for when appointments are running behind or when patients are late.

- Keep fees fair and competitive.
- Make a policy on financial arrangements and stick to it.
- Provide more than the patient expects. Examples: free coffee, current magazines, fresh flowers, toys for children, television, free monthly drawings, and tours for patients' friends and families.

These, and other topics, will be addressed in a *Standard Office Procedure Manual* to be implemented by all office personnel in accordance with the Total Quality Management philosophy.

Differentiation. If an office can offer something that few others have, a *uniqueness of practice*, it will attract a significantly greater percentage of the potential target population than without that uniqueness. Here are some ideas for AllYear Chiropractic:

- Hours: Make visiting the practice convenient for the patients. Examples of special considerations may include: Saturday hours, evening and early morning hours, lunch hours, etc.. The cost might include extra staff (twenty hours per week), $120. Evaluation of the effectiveness of this approach will include a determination of the cost-effectiveness of the odd hours, as well as the additional stress placed, thereby, on the doctors and staff members.
- Events: Sponsoring a luncheon, a Khorey-league team, or a radio show might provide a doctor and the practice with exposure not seen by most clinicians.
- Slogan/Logo: A strong slogan and logo will not only attract patients, it will familiarize the general public with the office. The slogan and logo will be pervasive. It will appear on all communications from the practice, including all business cards, stationery, and advertisements, newsletters, and so forth. At the moment of writing this plan, the following logo and slogan have been adopted:

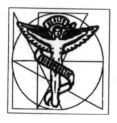

ALLYEAR CHIROPRACTIC
Quality Alternative Health Care
Year Around

Referrals. Staff referrals are a compliment by the employees to the practice. Rewarding such support seems appropriate. AllYear Chiropractic will give incentives for staff referrals. These will be provided prior to the end of the year at a special holiday "appreciation" dinner and party. To assist staff members in producing referrals, each member will have his or her own business cards and stationery. This will cost approximately thirty dollars per year, in addition to the bonuses. Patient referrals shall not go unnoticed either. A thank-you card will be sent to each patient who refers someone. In addition, one regular office visit will be offered to the referring patient at no charge. This cost is negligible, and is offset by the income generated by the new patient. This will be standard procedure.

Principals and Advisors

The success of a new organization depends to a large extent on the skills, energy and efforts of the principals, staff, and advisors involved in the endeavor. While initially the staff of AllYear Chiropractic will consist of the principals; future staff selection will appraise the attitude, skills, experience, and energy of the individuals under consideration. A synopsis of the two principals and their major advisors follows.

Bruce Player, D.C.

Bruce graduated from Logan College of Chiropractic (St. Louis, Missouri) with a Doctorate of Chiropractic on April 16, 1994, after a distinguished and active college career. Bruce's Chiropractic qualifications include Activator Methods, Cox Technique, Diversified Technique, and Basic Technique. He maintained a high academic standing while pursuing many collegiate, professional, and community activities. He was a member of Chi Rho Sigma (a coeducational, professional fraternity) from October, 1991 until graduation. He served as its vice-president and later president from November 1991 until April 1993, and was its representative to the Logan Student Doctor's Council (student government). In addition, Bruce served as class vice-president for four semesters and as class education coordinator for two semesters. He is a member of the World Congress of Chiropractic Students and served in the following capacities: delegate, 1992 Convention at New York Chiropractic College; fundraising chairman, 1993 Convention at Logan Chiropractic College; 1993 W.C.C.S. Convention in St. Louis—head delegate, Logan College. He holds the following professional memberships: World Congress of Chiropractic Students Alumni, American Chiropractic Association (A.C.A.), Missouri State Chiropractic Association, Logan College of Chiropractic Alumni Association. Future post-graduate educational goals include qualifying as a Certified Chiropractic Sports Physician (a three-year program); Diplomate in Nutrition (five years). Bruce's personality, experiences, and clinical skills will be material factors in the success of the practice.

James T. Swanson

Jim will graduate from Logan College of Chiropractic on August 6, 1994, with a Doctorate of Chiropractic. He will receive his license to practice in the State of Missouri within days of graduation. Until that time Jim will perform examinations and physical therapy in the practice under the supervision of Dr. Player. Jim's chiropractic qualifications include Applied Kinesiology, Diversified Technique, and Basic Technique. He maintained a high academic standing while pursuing the following collegiate, professional, and community activities: class secretary; class vice-president; President Student Doctors Council (student government) from July 1993 until April 1994; president, Logan Student Chapter of the American Chiropractic Association. In this latter capacity, Jim was elected and served for one year as national legislative vice-chairman, responsible for organizing and mobilizing students at thirteen chiropractic colleges in response to legislative proposals and actions. Prior to entering Logan, Jim served with honor and distinction in a number of public safety and emergency response agencies in supervisory capacities in New York and California. His experience in managing paid and volunteer workers, planning and supervising disaster response exercises, and public communication will be a material factor in the success of the practice.

A. Fuller Jurist, Jr., J.D.

Andy will assist the practice with the legal and tax matters relating to the corporate startup and the operation of the practice. He received his law degree from St. Louis University and holds a Masters (L.L.M.) in tax law from Washington University. As a partner in the firm of Freund, Jurist, Komen & Freund, P.C., his primary area of practice is corporate, tax, and securities law. Andy has been a speaker, moderator, and lecturer at a number of professional seminars and institutes, including some sponsored by the St. Louis Metropolitan Bar Association and the National Business Institute. Besides his active membership in professional organizations, including the American Bar Association, Missouri Bar Association, and the St. Louis Metropolitan Bar Association, Andy serves on the board of directors of a number of local civic and charitable organizations. His experience, knowledge, skill, and insight are additional factors for success for this new endeavor.

Rudolf P. Vrugtman, M.B.A

Rudi will assist the practice in the business management and financial areas. Over the last two decades, he has owned and operated a small business (R & R Financial Services, Inc.), and advised numerous businesses, including health-care firms. He is a faculty member at Logan College of Chiropractic, St. Louis College of Health Careers, and National-Louis University, teaching business and finance courses. In addition, he is a frequent lecturer at seminars and courses at other health-care education institutions. Besides his professional designations, he holds an M.B.A in Finance from Webster University and has many hours of post graduate credit from Washington University in taxation, accounting, finance, and business management. He is a published author and co-author of two textbooks for business courses in the health care environment. He operates a thriving consulting business which advises approximately thirty-five chiropractic physicians across the country, in addition to other commercial establishments. Taxes, finance, and business management clearly are his strengths. His skill and expertise is an additional factor predicting success for this new endeavor.

John D. Smith, D.C.

Dr. Smith owns and operates two successful practices in south St. Louis. He holds a Doctorate of Chiropractic from Logan College of Chiropractic, and has served the community for more then twenty years as a physician. John's chiropractic qualifications include Activator Methods, Diversified Technique, and Basic Technique. He has completed post-graduate programs in radiology, nutrition, and disability impairment rating. Besides active professional and community involvement John strongly supports professional education. For more then fifteen years his offices have been intern sites for Logan College, where seniors complete their clinical education. His *Standard Office Procedures Manual* and *Standard Treatment Protocols* are widely accepted and are utilized by chiropractic physicians nationwide. John's clinical and business insights and experience will be major additional factors in the success of the practice.

Chiropractic's Position in Health Care

Chiropractic is a health-care specialty utilizing conservative, non-invasive care to correct and prevent injuries and illness. Most chiropractors specialize in musculo-skeletal symptoms, many emphasize and teach preventative care. Ergonomics, the study of the human body in the work environment, is heavily populated with chiropractors and orthopedists. Recent studies indicate that chiropractic care is the most cost-effective approach to musculo-skeletal dysfunction and is the preferred treatment for many worker's compensation and accidental bodily injuries. Many sports injuries frequently respond best to chiropractic care.

Nationwide, there are approximately thirty-five thousand chiropractors, nearly five hundred of whom practice in the Greater St. Louis Metropolitan area. In the United States there are thirteen chiropractic colleges annually graduating approximately three thousand physicians. This rate is slightly higher than a replacement rate. Chiropractic is becoming more accepted as a health-care branch in this country, though it has yet to achieve the level of acceptance it has long held in Europe and the Pacific Rim countries. Chiropractic education, today, is on an equal quality and intensiveness level with medical and osteopathic education, in certain bio-mechanic, pharmacological and nutritional concentration areas, it is in fact advanced. This is definitely the case for business education, where Logan is in the lead, not just in chiropractic education, but in all health-care education. Logan graduates have been exposed to more business thoughts, concepts, and procedures then any other physicians at graduation.

The last complete study to develop a financial profile of chiropractors in the United States was done by the American Chiropractic Association in 1985. It is the feeling of the advisors to the practice that this information is now outdated. Therefore, the following information was developed by the advisors from their own client files of St. Louis area offices. A "typical" St. Louis chiropractor will need three to four years to develop the practice to a mature state. This is partially the result of the third-party reimbursement and payment factors in the industry. Delays of payment for fees of six to eight weeks are common, while "fee cutting" is becoming an occasional factor. These factors are being aggravated by "managed care" organizations such as HMOs and PPOs, an increasing factor in the health-care industry. While those organizations have not yet focused on the chiropractors, it appears to be only a matter of time before they do. Additional delays can be expected if a patient's case involves litigation, as will occur in some worker's compensation and many accidental bodily injury situations. The "average" St. Louis chiropractor can expect to generate approximately $150,000–$400,000 in annual fees per physician, on approximately two hundred to three hundred patient office visits per month. While both of these statistics are below those of medical and osteopathic physicians in the St. Louis area, the "gap" has been closing over the last decade. A 92–95 percent collection ratio is common. On a cash accounting basis, overhead can be expected to run in the 30–40 percent range, depending mostly on the size and location of the office and the physicians and the effective and efficient use of staff. Common after-tax income to the chiropractor is in the $60,000–$150,000 range for a physician in a mature practice.

Business Format and Responsibilities of the Principals

Player-Swanson Chiropractic, P. C. will be a Missouri corporation with a charter issued under the Professional Corporation laws, as required by the Code of Ethics of the Missouri State Chiropractors Association. Initially, only Dr. Bruce Player will be a shareholder, as state law requires. A stock option will be issued to Jim Swanson to require him to purchase 50 percent of the corporation upon his receipt of a Missouri chiropractors license. An agreement has been executed between the two principals and Jim Swanson has contributed 50 percent of the initial capital of the corporation. This is carried on the books of the corporation as a loan, until the time the stock option is exercised. It is the intent of the principals to be considered as equally liable and responsible from the inception of the operations, notwithstanding the legal environment. Neither principal would have considered starting a practice from scratch, in the manner here described, without being assured of the support and assistance of the other principal. It is anticipated that Dr. Swanson will be "legal" to practice, and thus exercise his stock option, around the middle of August 1994.

A buy-sell agreement is currently being prepared by legal counsel and will cover all contingencies: death, disability, and termination/retirement. The agreement will be funded using appropriate life and disability insurance policies. Initially, termination/retirement buyout (not anticipated to occur for quite a few years) will be accomplished through a series of personal notes; as soon as the practice is past the initial startup phase, funding through deferred compensation agreements will be initiated.

Basic agreement has been reached between the principals on the division of day-to-day business responsibilities. Certain business decisions will be made only by mutual consent: those dealing with major financial matters, all legal matters, standard operating procedures and standard treatment protocols, employment and termination of paraprofessional and professional employees and their training, as well as the selection and employment of advisors.

Cash-flow Projections

As in all business startup situations, cash flow is crucial for survival and must, therefore, be tightly controlled. The principals and advisors are aware of the largely arbitrary value of "best estimate" forecasts and the high uncertainty factor involved in projections. Borrowing from the capital budgeting techniques, sensitivity analysis was used. Cash-flow projections were developed using three scenarios: (B) Most Likely—Best Estimate, (A) Less Likely—Worst Case, and, (C) Less Likely—Best Case. Probabilities were assigned to the three scenarios as follows: (A) 25 percent, (B) 50 percent, (C) 25 percent. Each scenario was developed independently of the others.

For the calendar year 1994 (and finished for a full fifty-two weeks, in order to develop a projection basis) cash inflow projections were calculated on a weekly basis. Factors used in the projection of revenue (cash basis) are: new patients attracted to the practice, standard treatment protocol, standard office visit fee schedule, assumed patient mix (10 percent cash, 50 percent health insurance, 20 percent personal injury and litigated worker's comp, and 15 percent other), average third-party payment delay (eight weeks). These cash inflows are then recapitulated on a monthly basis to be merged with the cash outflow projections. Thus cash deficits can be projected on a monthly basis. The scenario B projections and the cumulative cash-flow graph is shown in the financial illustrations. Annual cash-flow projections for 1995 and 1996 are displayed as well for Scenario B. Details of all calculations are available upon request.

While these initial projections have a high degree of risk attached to them, it is the intent of the principals and advisors to update them on a regular basis (bimonthly) as experience is gained with actual operations. In this manner, it is anticipated that cash-flow control will become a tool used to assure survival, which in the first three years of operation equates to success.

Pro Forma Balance Sheets

The pro forma balance sheets, as shown in the financial statement section of the appendix, are presented in the format of generally accepted accounting procedures. Because of this, a few items must be noted to translate the statements to the real-world situation.

Cash in bank has been used as a balancing account other than in the opening balance sheet. Operating financial policy will be to keep a minimal balance in a corporate checking account and to maintain the remainder in a money-market type of fund. Of course, negotiation with a financial institution for the required loans may alter this plan. Inventory will consist of small quantities of orthopedic supports and implements together with nutritional supplements and vitamins for sale to patients. Accounts receivable will be mainly from third-party payors. Normal operating experience in the St. Louis area indicates a forty-five to sixty days to cash period.

Furniture and equipment values indicate the value of both office and clinic equipment to be acquired. A complete detailed list is available on request. Depreciation is calculated based on election of ten thousand dollars expensing (section 179) in calendar year one and depreciation using the five year (half year convention) MACRS table. Amortization of leasehold improvements over the seventy-two-month lease is included.

Security deposits show a return of the deposits from the utility companies during the second full year of operation. The real-estate deposit is expected to remain for the full seventy-two months of the lease. Organization expenses are being written off over the statutory seven years.

Taxes payable indicate an arbitrary amount owed for payroll taxes on December 31 of each year. Equipment notes or leases show a payoff over sixty months with a moratorium or "contract payment" token amount during three or six months. Telephone equipment ($1,500) is on a thirty-six-month financial lease from SouthWestern Bell (at an imputed interest rate of 6 percent). Detailed amortization schedules are available upon request. Working capital balances are taken from Scenario B—the most likely cash-flow projections.

For certain tax and future financial flexibility purposes, legal capitalization has been kept to an absolute minimum. *For lending purposes the value of the loans from officers is in reality a capital or equity account.* It is anticipated that income tax returns will be prepared on a cash accounting basis, rather then an accrual basis. The principals may elect not to receive a salary during the first year to year and a half of operations. The main effect of this will be to reduce payroll and personal and corporate income taxes payable, and thus save overall cash flow. Both principals will require some cash from operation to support their families. It is anticipated that at no time (while debt financing is in existence) the "real equity" will be negative. A recalculation of equity is shown below.

Restated Pro Forma Balance Sheet —Equity and Debt Positions

	June 1994	1994	1995	1996
Real Equity: Total equity plus loan from officers	$16,000	$10,671	$27,223	$47,873
Real Debt: Long-term debt minus loan from officers	$26,086	$39,368	$35,970	$27,677
True Equity Ratio (to total assets)	38%	21%	42%	62%

Milestones and Critical Factors

As indicated earlier in this paper, opening day of the practice is anticipated to be June 15, 1994. A real-estate lease has been signed by the principals, the lease deposit paid. The lease is a three-year lease with a three-year option to renew. The lease is effective May 1, 1994, with $ 0 rent due for the first three months. Thereafter, monthly lease payments will be $1,100 together with the $218.16 monthly common charges. Utilities are the responsibility of the corporation. Should there be reason to postpone the effective date of the lease (licensing or financing situations), the landlord has verbally agreed to a deferral until August 1, 1994, at the latest.

The plans for this endeavor depend to an extent on the licensure of Mr. Swanson as Chiropractor. Licensing requirements in the state of Missouri are: graduation from an accredited chiropractic school, passing of certain portions of National Board of Chiropractic examinations, and passing of the State Board of Chiropractic examination. Upon completion of these requirements issuance of the license by the State Board of Healing Arts is a matter of paperwork normally completed in three to five days. Mr. Swanson is expected to graduate from Logan on August 6, 1994. While there is a possibility of delay in this, it is minimal, as he has successfully completed all required class work and is well into completion of the clinical stage. His performance in this phase is exemplary, as reported unofficially by his supervising professors. He has passed the requisite National Boards and expects to be able to pass the State Boards in June 1994. Thus licensure is expected by the middle of August 1994. Dr. Player is fully licensed to practice chiropractic in Missouri.

Construction inside the leased space is expected to take less than two weeks. Currently, selection of a contractor is being finalized and construction is expected to start in the middle of May 1994. Delivery of the required office and clinic furniture and equipment is a matter of days following the issuance of a purchase order. The purchase orders have been prepared and are being held pending final financing arrangements. Only the x-ray equipment will require installation, to be completed in less then one day. The x-ray equipment supplier has assured that this will be accomplished within one week of delivery of the equipment. Should there be an unforeseen delay, arrangements have been made with the Montgomery Clinic of Logan College (four miles removed from the practice) to provide the necessary services there. While this may inconvenience some early patients, it is not expected to be necessary or to be a major obstacle.

Finally, health care in the United States is in a state of change. State and national health-care proposals are being considered in the legislatures. Predicting the outcome of these deliberations is impossible at this stage, however, it appears that chiropractic will remain a viable health care profession. With or without changes in law, third-party reimbursement rules and procedures will change in the next few years. While some of the changes may negatively influence the cash-flow position of health-care providers, they are not expected to endanger the success of this endeavor materially.

Financing Proposal

Request is hereby made to arrange the debt financing required for the successful launch of the practice. Two alternatives are suggested:

A. Bank financing for the complete package as follows:
1. A five-year term loan for the acquisition of the required equipment in the amount of approximately twenty-six thousand dollars.
2. If possible, inclusion in the above term loan of the approximately five thousand dollars required for the lease-hold improvement construction (increases the amount to approximately thirty-one thousand dollars).
3. Establishing a working capital line of credit of no more then thirty thousand dollars available for drawing until December 31, 1995.
4. At that time, the principals anticipate combining the two loans into one note with a fixed or variable interest rate and a three- to five-year amortization schedule.
5. Collateral offered are the equipment and furniture to be acquired, assignment of the accounts receivable, collateral assignment of adequate life and disability income policies on each of the two principals.
6. Establishment of a long-term banking relationship for business and personal transactions of the principals.

B. Bank financing for working capital only as follows:
1. Establishing a working capital line of credit of no more than thirty thousand dollars, available for drawing until December 31, 1995.
2. At that time, the principals anticipate changing to a note with a fixed or variable interest rate and a three- to five-year amortization schedule.
3. Collateral offered are assignment of the accounts receivable, collateral assignment of adequate life and disability income policies on each of the two principals.
4. Establishment of a long-term banking relationship for business and personal transactions of the principals.

Financial Illustrations

Cash-flow Projections 1994 to 1996

Cash-flow Graph

Pro Forma Balance Sheets, Inception to 12/31/96

Monthly Cash-flow Projections 1994

Cash-flow Projections Graph 1994

Patient Office Visit Projections Graph 1994

Cash-Flow Projections
Player & Swanson Chiropractic PC

	1994	1995	1996
New Patients OV	67	180	252
Return Patients OV	755	2096	2725
Established Patients OV	103	85	43
Total OVs	925	2361	3019
Beginning Cash from Operations	$0	($11,036)	($12,352)
Total Fees	$46,205	$117,127	$158,122
Established Patients	$4,841	$2,550	$1,275
Total Collections	$25,263	$119,677	$159,397
Staff Salaries & PRT	$0	$12,000	$20,000
Rent	$9,663	$16,572	$16,572
Utilities	$1,725	$2,220	$2,331
Phone	$870	$1,500	$1,725
Office Supplies	$2,000	$3,800	$4,560
Clinic Supplies	$1,025	$2,200	$2,530
Dues & Subscriptions	$850	$1,075	$1,129
Advertising	$1,000	$2,500	$2,125
Equipment Lease (P&I)	$3,945	$7,740	$7,740
Malpractice Insurance	$1,125	$2,400	$3,000
General Insurance	$2,030	$3,600	$3,780
Legal & Accounting	$1,875	$2,900	$2,900
Taxes & Licenses	$300	$900	$900
Seminars & Education	$1,200	$2,400	$3,600
Laundry & Uniforms	$500	$675	$725
Interest	$1,866	$3,000	$2,000
Bank Expense	$275	$425	$475
Miscellaneous	$6,050	$8,086	$8,414
Dr. Draws/Loans	$3,200	$42,000	($45,200)
Dr. Salaries & PRT	$0	$0	$100,000
Total Expenses	$36,299	$115,993	$139,306
Debt Service	$0	$5,000	$10,000
Net Annual Cash flow	($11,036)	($1,316)	$10,091
Cummulative CF from operations	($11,036)	($12,352)	($2,261)

Cash-flow Projections 1994 to 1996

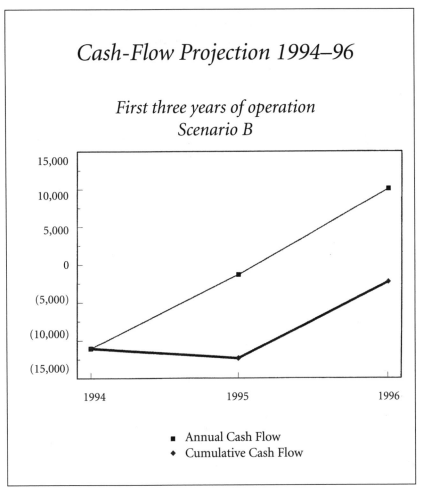

Cash-flow Graph

Pro Forma Balance Sheets
Player & Swanson Chiropractic PC

	Opening June 94	Year End 1994	Year End 1995	Year End 1996
Current Assets				
Cash in Bank	$3,125	$2,500	$4,000	$10,000
Inventory	$250	$250	$250	$250
Accounts Receivable	$0	$25,783	$47,500	$60,250
Total Current Assets	$3,375	$28,533	$51,750	$70,500
Fixed Assets				
Furniture & Equipment	$31,311	$31,311	$31,311	$31,311
Leasehold Improvements	$5,000	$5,000	$5,000	$5,000
Fixed Assets at Cost	$36,311	$36,311	$36,311	$36,311
Accumulated Depreciation	$0	$15,762	$25,182	$31,232
Net Fixed Assets	$36,311	$20,549	$11,129	$5,079
Other Assets				
Security Deposits	$1,400	$1,400	$1,100	$1,100
Organization Expenses	$1,000	$857	$714	$571
Total Other Assets	$2,400	$2,257	$1,814	$1,671
Total Assets	$42,086	$51,339	$64,693	$77,250
Liabilities and Equity				
Liabilities				
Current Liabilities				
Accounts Payable	$0	$0	$0	$0
Taxes Payable	$0	$300	$500	$700
Total Current Liabilities	$0	$300	$500	$700
Long-Term Liabilities				
Equipment Notes or Leases	$26,086	$28,332	$23,618	$17,677
Working Capital Bank Note	$0	$11,036	$12,352	$10,000
Loan from Officers	$15,000	$15,399	$16,448	$30,800
Total Long-Term Liabilities	$41,086	$54,767	$52,418	$58,477
Total Liabilities	$41,086	$55,067	$52,918	$59,177
Equity				
Common Stock @ $1 par	$200	$200	$200	$200
Paid in Capital	$800	$800	$800	$800
Retained Earnings	$0	($4,728)	$10,775	$17,073
Total Equity	$1,000	($3,728)	$11,775	$18,073
Total Liabilities and Equity	$42,086	$51,339	$64,693	$77,250

Pro Forma Balance Sheets, Inception to 12/31/96

Initial Cash-Flow Projections—Player & Swanson Chiropractic PC
Scenario B

	Jan	Feb	Mar	Apr	May	Jun	Jul	Aug	Sep	Oct	Nov	Dec	1994
New Patients OV	0	0	0	0	2	4	7	6	18	11	13	6	67
Return Pts OV	0	0	0	0	0	30	68	72	146	145	141	153	755
Established Pts OV	0	0	0	0	7	14	17	14	17	14	12	8	103
Total OVs	0	0	0	0	9	48	92	92	181	170	166	167	925
Beginning Cash	$0.00	$0.00	($210.00)	($2,280.00)	($6,595.99)	($9,159.72)	($10,170.29)	($11,110.36)	($13,378.38)	($12,526.74)	($12,299.42)	($12,056.60)	$0.00
Total Fees	$0.00	$0.00	$0.00	$0.00	$320.00	$2050.00	$4,316.00	$4,344.00	$9,742.00	$8,575.00	$8,707.00	$8,151.00	$46,205.00
Established Patients	$0.00	$0.00	$0.00	$0.00	$329.00	$658.00	$799.00	$658.00	$799.00	$658.00	$564.00	$376.00	$4,841.00
Total Collections	$0.00	$0.00	$0.00	$0.00	$425.00	$1,273.00	$2,337.74	$2,492.97	$4,664.03	$4,306.90	$4,833.60	$4,929.84	$25,263.08
Rent	$0.00	$0.00	$1,100.00	$218.16	$218.16	$218.16	$1,318.16	$1,318.16	$1,318.16	$1,318.16	$1318.16	$1,318.16	$9,663.44
Utilities	$0.00	$0.00	$0.00	$300.00	$150.00	$150.00	$200.00	$225.00	$225.00	$175.00	$150.00	$150.00	$1,725.00
Phone	$0.00	$50.00	$50.00	$100.00	$90.00	$90.00	$90.00	$90.00	$90.00	$90.00	$90.00	$90.00	$870.00
Office Supplies	$0.00	$0.00	$300.00	$150.00	$300.00	$300.00	$150.00	$150.00	$150.00	$150.00	$150.00	$150.00	$2,000.00
Clinic Supplies	$0.00	$0.00	$0.00	$250.00	$250.00	$75.00	$75.00	$75.00	$75.00	$75.00	$75.00	$75.00	$1,025.00
Dues & Subs	$0.00	$0.00	$150.00	$150.00	$75.00	$225.00	$100.00	$50.00	$25.00	$25.00	$25.00	$25.00	$850.00
Advertising	$0.00	$0.00	$0.00	$500.00	$0.00	$0.00	$0.00	$500.00	$0.00	$0.00	$0.00	$0.00	$1,000.00
Equipment Lease	$0.00	$0.00	$0.00	$645.00	$25.00	$25.00	$25.00	$645.00	$645.00	$645.00	$645.00	$645.00	$3,945.00
Malpractice Ins	$0.00	$0.00	$0.00	$225.00	$0.00	$0.00	$225.00	$225.00	$0.00	$225.00	$225.00	$0.00	$1,125.00
General Insurance	$0.00	$0.00	$0.00	$430.00	$200.00	$200.00	$200.00	$200.00	$200.00	$200.00	$200.00	$200.00	$2,030.00
Legal & Accounting	$0.00	$125.00	$125.00	$325.00	$425.00	$125.00	$125.00	$125.00	$125.00	$125.00	$125.00	$125.00	$1,875.00
Taxes & Licenses	$0.00	$0.00	$0.00	$100.00	$100.00	$25.00	$0.00	$100.00	$0.00	$0.00	$0.00	$0.00	$300.00
Seminars & Educ	$0.00	$0.00	$0.00	$0.00	$500.00	$300.00	$0.00	$0.00	$0.00	$0.00	$400.00	$0.00	$1,200.00
Laundry & Uniforms	$0.00	$0.00	$0.00	$100.00	$50.00	$50.00	$50.00	$50.00	$50.00	$50.00	$50.00	$50.00	$500.00
Interest	$0.00	$0.00	$0.00	$28.50	$82.45	$119.81	$148.35	$189.33	$248.84	$296.49	$347.49	$404.87	$1,866.13
Bank Expense	$0.00	$0.00	$0.00	$75.00	$25.00	$25.00	$25.00	$25.00	$25.00	$25.00	$25.00	$25.00	$275.00
Miscellaneous	$0.00	$35.00	$345.00	$719.33	$498.12	$380.59	$546.30	$793.50	$635.40	$679.93	$765.13	$651.61	$6,049.91
Dr. Draws /Loans	$0.00	$0.00	$0.00	$0.00	$0.00	$0.00	$0.00	$400.00	$400.00	$600.00	$800.00	$1,000.00	$3,200.00
Total Expenses	$0.00	$210.00	$2,070.00	$4,315.99	$2,988.73	$2,283.56	$3,277.82	$4,760.98	$3,812.40	$4,079.58	$4,590.78	$3,909.64	$36,299.49
Monthly Cash Flow	$0.00	($210.00)	($2,070.00)	($4,315.99)	($2,563.73)	($1,010.56)	($940.07)	($2,268.02)	$851.64	$227.32	$242.82	$1,020.20	($11,036.41)
Ending Cash	$0.00	($210.00)	($2,280.00)	($6,595.99)	($9,159.72)	($10,170.29)	($11,110.36)	($13,378.38)	($12,526.74)	($12,299.42)	($12,056.60)	($11,036.41)	($11,036.41)

Monthly Cash-flow Projections 1994

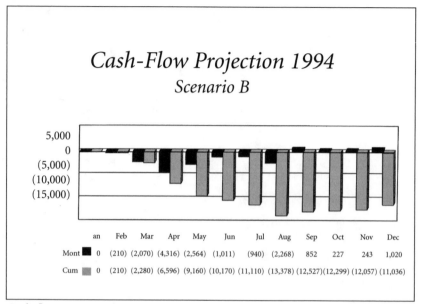

Cash-flow Projections Graph 1994

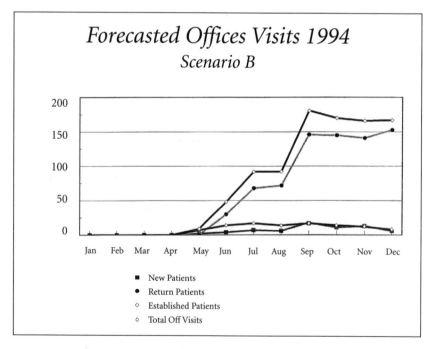

Patient Office Visit Projections Graph 1994

Appendix H
Business Plan and Loan Proposal—Buying a Practice

This appendix illustrates the form and components of a business plan and loan proposal for buying a practice. The primary differences between this business plan and the previous plan for a start up practice are the presence of existing patients, the resultant cash flow, and the financial capability of the seller to provide loan money for the purchase.

Freeman Chiropractic

BUSINESS PLAN AND LOAN PROPOSAL

Freeman Chiropractic
Your caregiver for better health

Business Plan: Freeman Chiropractic

Executive Summary
Marketing Plan
    Established Patients
    Personal Marketing
    Promotion
    Customer-oriented Management and Customer Relations
Principals and Advisors
    Hendrik Freeman, D.C.
    Mitsy Lawyer, J.D.
    Rudolf P. Vrugtman, M.B.A
    John D. White, D.C.
Chiropractic's Position in Health Care
Business Format and Responsibilities of the Principals
Financial Forecasts
    Cash-flow Projections
    Pro Forma Balance Sheets
Milestones and Critical Factors
Financing Proposal

Business Plan
Freeman Chiropractic

Executive Summary

Freeman Chiropractic is the trade name for a Chiropractic Professional Corporation in organization. The incorporator is Dr. Hendrik Freeman, who will have the charter application filed within days of receiving his license to practice in the State of Indiana. It is anticipated that Freeman will be open for the treatment of the first patients on March 5, 1996. The practice will be located at 4515 Main Street at the intersection of Main Street and Twenty-second Avenue, in west Franklin County.

It is intended that the corporation, following the initial meeting, be owned by Dr. Freeman. This business plan has been prepared for internal management use and to familiarize the reader and potential lender with the plans and projections.

The corporation will buy assets from the practice of Dr. Seller, currently operating at 4515 Main. To assure that established patients will feel welcome to discuss their concerns with the new doctor, Dr. Seller will remain as part of the practice for approximately three months after Dr. Freeman takes ownership. Compensation for Dr. Seller for this period is included in the purchase price of the practice.

The startup process for any professional endeavor is characterized by two main factors. First, no matter how capable the management is from a clinical or business perspective, a period of negative cash flow exists in the beginning. Professional practices have high fixed costs relative to the variable costs per patient. Therefore, while the patient office visit count is low, cash flow will be negative. Second, the doctor-patient relationship is based on personal trust. This means that marketing strategies depending on advertising to draw threshold traffic may not be effective. This practice will rely on more appropriate marketing strategies that will develop long-term patient relationships. These strategies will, by their very nature, result in a slower initial growth in office visits, but should in the long run prove more profitable.

In this endeavor, cash flow and marketing will be the crucial factors in the first few years. The principal believes that he has, with the assistance of his advisors, developed plans and strategies to deal effectively with the pitfalls of starting a professional office. Using currently accepted financial measures, they expect to invest 38 percent equity at inception. The equity ratio will fall slightly during the startup phase to a low of 21 percent after a year and a half of operations, then quickly rebound to more then 60 percent after three years. Though opening day is still nearly two months away, initial marketing efforts have been started and will be the primary concern of principal and advisors for the next three years.

Financing will need to be arranged for the endeavor to be successful. A loan of twenty-five thousand dollars will be sought in the form of a term loan for acquisition of equipment and initial supplies. In addition, a working capital line of credit of thirty thousand will be sought to assist in surviving the above described negative cash flow. At the time of writing this plan, two leasing companies have committed to provide the term financing.

Marketing Plan

Because of the nature of the relationship between doctor and patient, a relationship of personal trust which takes time to develop, the marketing strategies described below emphasize the two required factors: time and personal contact. While some advertising type strategies will be employed, these will concentrate on name recognition and image development rather then the more immediate "action generating" style intended only to develop threshold traffic. In the experience of the advisors, patients drawn by threshold traffic advertising do not fit the target population characteristics of this practice, as they are primarily motivated by cut-rate fees and discount promotions, rather than quality health care provided with an eye on quality of life for the patient. Initial marketing efforts have already yielded a small number of "promised" patients at opening.

Established Patients

The acquisition of Dr. Genie Seller's patient files will be material in generating the cash flow projected in the appendices. Dr. Seller has owned and operated the practice for a total of fifteen years, of which the last eight were in the current location. This is also the proposed location for Freeman Chiropractic, P.C. Dr. Seller has excellent relations with her patients, many of them having received care at her office for a long time. Dr. Seller practices in her office five days per week and sees an average of four hundred patient office visits per week. Dr. Freeman intends to keep the operation of the office as close to the same as possible in order to allow the established patients the comfort level required to adjust to a new doctor. Projections include an assumption of a loss of established patients (25 percent) at a level judged appropriate for the change in physician.

To assure Dr. Freeman of appropriate information about the feelings and attitudes of the existing patients, he has arranged for Mr. James Loew, of Fayette, to host a series of focus group sessions with patients jointly selected by Drs. Freeman and Seller. Focus group discussions will center on the desires of the patients for appropriate operations and quality delivery of care during the ownership transition period.

Personal Marketing

The principal is currently engaged in activities designed to develop local community awareness of the practice and himself. Dr. Freeman has arranged to be guest speaker at a number of service organizations and frequently visits on a low-key basis with employers and business owners in the target market area. During these conversations he presents the recent Manga study results on the efficiency of chiropractic care in the worker's compensation area. He also discusses the well-established preventative care results provided by chiropractic care. In addition, he reviews the results he obtained with worker's compensation claims while in practice in the St. Louis area. Chiropractic has been found to be more cost-effective and to produce lower levels of time lost then other modes of treatment for a large variety of worker's compensation injuries. Dr. Freeman has used the patient education materials and systems developed by BackTalk Systems, Inc. of Colorado Springs effectively in his prior practice experience and expects to continue to do so. Specific strategies to be employed:

Public speaking. The practice of speaking in front of groups and organizations increases visibility and recognition of the practice and its principals. It is almost required in today's health-care environment, besides, Dr. Freeman is comfortable and effective in group communication situations. The costs involved in doing this is strictly time and energy. Preparation is required and might steal time from other marketing tools, however, no other approach has shown the positive results from a cost-benefit point of view.

Community involvement. Any business organization that receives support from its community is obligated to "return" the favor by supporting involvement of its employees and owners. The principal intends to provide an example for future staff members by active involvement in selected organizations. While there certainly is a marketing angle to this involvement, selection of the organizations to become active in will be based primarily on personal preferences and philosophies. The costs are a time factor and relatively small membership and meeting dues. A list of possible involvement for the principals follows.

- St. Mark's Lutheran School PTO
- Managing children's sports teams (basketball little league)
- Sponsoring and managing adult leagues (bowling)
- Health-club memberships

Promotion

Advertising. This will include initial and annual open-house ads, wellness programs, image programs developing chiropractic and practice recognition in the community, and the like. Discounts and other fee-reducing advertising, typically, is not cost-effective, as it draws the wrong kind of patient. Copies of advertisements may be mailed an average of four times per year to a select part of the target population with an appropriate cover letter. The outcome measurement of this particular marketing strategy is deceiving. While few new patients will be developed as a direct result of this route, existing patients may be encouraged to stay and may even feel comfortable referring others. The name recognition resulting from this effort should be invaluable in the long run.

Newsletters. A newsletter will not generate immediate new patient traffic. Instead, it is a strategy designed to develop image and name recognition and, if properly targeted, may cause "centers of influence" to refer patients. It may also maintain existing patients. To inform a target population of the status of the clinic and chiropractic is the primary objective. Patient education ultimately leads to referrals. Three quality newsletters a year will be the original goal. At five hundred mailed, the overall cost will be $930 yearly.

Allied Health Care Network. This network will be formed by Freeman Chiropractic. Its members would include interested doctors of various specialties, attorneys, and so forth. The main purpose is to provide a referral source to and from Freeman Chiropractic. The costs would include mailing, luncheons, and telephone fees, and should not exceed three hundred dollars per year.

Dr. Freeman has become a member of the Business Referral Network of Franklin County. This organizations consists of twenty-five local business owners and professionals who assist their clients in referring them to other professionals and businesses they require. The club meets every Wednesday for lunch.

Customer-Oriented Management and Patient Relations

Total Quality Management. This concept will be the theme of all activity of the practice. Quality is defined as responsiveness to the needs of the clientele. Regardless of how long a practice has been in existence, as long as it is continuously trying to improve, it will grow. Regular staff meetings will suggest operational and other factors requiring attention. Often, the patients will tell the staff members things they would never say to the doctor. Open and honest communication with employees will develop more ideas and suggestions than ever thought possible. In many chiropractic offices the progress of a patient is re-evaluated after eight or ten visits. At Freeman Chiropractic, the practice will be evaluated by each patient, each time the patient is clinically re-evaluated for care, thus creating two-way communication. Suggestions from these evaluations will be discussed at following staff meetings and, if appropriate, change in standard operating procedures or standard treatment protocol will be initiated. Costs are minimal (almost zero). Expected results would include a health-care office designed by patients.

Office Appearance. A professional appearance will suggest such thoughts as serious, successful, proud, compliance. To achieve this the staff must picture what the average patient perceives a friendly office to be. Cleanliness is a prerequisite. A dirty office does not denote health. Brightness is important, especially for people in pain and depression. Interesting wall decor might give an office a certain uniqueness. And clean, well-dressed staff is crucial for positive patients relations. Cleaning costs could vary, but might be estimated for five hours per week at six dollars per hour; yearly maintenance/decoration costs would be incurred in routine budget and lease arrangements.

Office Policies. Subtleties often represent the difference between a referral practice and a nonreferral practice; the details are that crucial. Many of these fall under the heading of general organization. Organization is expected in a professional practice and quality in organization becomes a marketing tool. Consideration for customers is likewise crucial. Showing patients that they are being considered is common sense, yet seldom done in the health-care industries. Some suggestions for Freeman Chiropractic include:

- Be sure the doctors are available when a patient wants to talk to them (i.e. telephone, letters).
- Have a fail-safe plan for when appointments are running behind or when patients are late.
- Keep fees fair and competitive.
- Make a policy on financial arrangements and stick to it, period!
- Provide more than the patient expects. Examples: Free coffee, current magazines, fresh flowers, toys for children, television, free monthly drawings, and tours for patients' friends and families.

These, and other topics, will be addressed in a *Standard Office Procedure Manual* to be implemented by all office personnel in accordance with the Total Quality Management philosophy.

Differentiation. If an office can offer something that few others have, a *uniqueness of practice,* it will attract a significantly greater percentage of the potential target population than without that uniqueness. Here are some ideas for Freeman Chiropractic:

- Hours: Make visiting the practice convenient for the patients. Examples of special considerations may include: Saturday hours, evening and early morning hours, lunch hours, etc. The cost might include extra staff (twenty hours per week), $120. Evaluation of the effectiveness of this approach will include a determination of the cost effectiveness of the odd hours, as well as the additional stress placed, thereby, on the doctors and staff members.

- Slogan/Logo: A slogan and logo will not only attract patients, it will familiarize the general public with the office. If done tastefully, there is little negative impact, yet much goodwill can be developed. The slogan and logo will be pervasive. It will appear on all communications from the practice, including all business cards, stationery, and advertisements, newsletters, and so forth. At the moment of writing this plan, the following logo and slogan have been adopted:

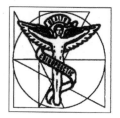

Freeman Chiropractic
Your caregiver for better health

- Events: Sponsoring a luncheon, a Khorey-league team, or a radio show might provide a doctor and the practice with exposure not seen by most clinicians.

Referrals. Staff referrals are a compliment by the employees to the practice. Rewarding such support seems appropriate. Freeman Chiropractic will give incentives for staff referrals. These will be provided prior to the end of the year at a special holiday "appreciation" dinner and party. To assist staff members in producing referrals, each member will have his or her own business cards and stationery. This will cost approximately thirty dollars per year, in addition to the bonuses. Patient referrals shall not go unnoticed either. A thank-you card will be sent to each patient who refers someone. In addition, one regular office visit will be offered to the referring patient at no charge. This cost is negligible, and is offset by the income generated by the new patient. This will be standard procedure.

Principal and Advisors

The success of a new organization depends to a large extent on the skills, energy and efforts of the principals, staff, and advisors involved in the endeavor. While initially the staff of Freeman Chiropractic will consist of the principal, Dr. Seller, the current front-desk assistant; future staff selection will appraise the attitude, skills, experience and energy of the individuals under consideration. A synopsis of the two principals and their major advisors follows.

Hendrik Freeman, D.C.

Harry graduated from Logan College of Chiropractic (St. Louis, Missouri) with a Doctorate of Chiropractic on April 14, 1993, after a distinguished and active career as a respiratory therapist in northern Michigan. Harry's Chiropractic qualifications include Gonstead, Cox, Diversified, and Logan Basic Techniques. In addition, Harry served as clinic coordinator and radiology red badge during his senior year. He is a member of the World Congress of Chiropractic Students and an advisory board member of the Logan Alumni Association. Harry practiced successfully in Chesterfield, Missouri, for nearly two years after graduation. He was an independent contractor in a chiropractic clinic owned and operated by a twenty-five year practitioner. He spent much of his time, when not treating patients, learning the business processes and operations from his mentor. Future postgraduate educational goals include qualifying as a Certified Chiropractic Sports Physician (a three-year program); Diplomate in Nutrition (five years). Harry's personality, experiences, and clinical skills will be material factors in the success of the practice.

Mitsy Lawyer, J.D.

Mitsy will assist the practice with the legal and tax matters relating to the corporate startup and the operation of the practice. She received her law degree from Indiana University and holds a Masters (LL.M.) in tax law from Ball State University. As a partner in the firm of James, Lawyer, and Dinger, P.C., her primary area of practice is corporate, tax and securities law. Mitsy has been a speaker, moderator, and lecturer at a number of professional seminars and institutes, including some sponsored by the Indiana State Bar Association and the National Business Institute. Besides her active membership in professional organizations, including the American Bar Association, and Indiana Bar Association, Mitsy serves on the boards of directors of a number of local civic and charitable organizations. Her experience, knowledge, skill and insight are additional factors for success for this new endeavor.

Rudolf P. Vrugtman, M.B.A.

Rudi will assist the practice in the business management and financial areas. Over the last two decades, he has owned and operated a small business (R & R Financial Services, Inc.), and advised numerous businesses, including health-care firms. He is a faculty member at Logan College of Chiropractic, St. Louis College of Health Careers, and National-Louis University, teaching business and finance courses. In addition, he is a frequent lecturer at seminars and courses at other health-care education institutions. Besides his professional designations, he holds an M.B.A. in Finance from Webster University and has many hours of post graduate credit from Washington University in taxation, accounting, finance, and business management. He is a published author and co-author of two textbooks for business courses in the health care environment. He operates a thriving consulting business which advises approximately thirty-five chiropractic physicians across the country, in addition to other commercial establishments. Taxes, finance, and business management clearly are his strengths. His skill and expertise are additional factors predicting success for this new endeavor.

John D. White, D.C.

Dr. White owns a successful practice in Indianapolis. He holds a Doctorate of Chiropractic from National College of Chiropractic, and has served the community for more then twenty years as a physician. John's chiropractic qualifications include Activator Methods, Diversified Technique, and Gonstead Technique. He has completed postgraduate programs in radiology, nutrition, and disability impairment rating. Besides active professional and community involvement John strongly supports professional education. For more then fifteen years his offices have been intern sites for National College, where seniors complete their clinical education. His *Standard Treatment Protocols* are widely accepted and are utilized by chiropractic physicians nationwide. John's clinical and business insights and experience will be major additional factors in the success of the practice.

Chiropractic's Position in Health Care

Chiropractic is a health-care specialty utilizing conservative, noninvasive care to correct and prevent injuries and illness. Most chiropractors specialize in musculo-skeletal symptoms, many emphasize and teach preventative care. Ergonomics, the study of the human body in the work environment, is heavily populated with chiropractors and orthopedists. Recent studies indicate that chiropractic care is the most cost-effective approach to musculo-skeletal dysfunction and is the preferred treatment for many worker's compensation and accidental bodily injuries. Many sports injuries frequently respond best to chiropractic care.

Nationwide there are approximately thirty-five thousand chiropractors, nearly five hundred of whom practice in the Greater Franklin Metropolitan area. In the United States there are thirteen chiropractic colleges annually graduating approximately three thousand physicians. This rate is slightly higher than a replacement rate. Chiropractic is becoming more accepted as a health-care branch in this country, though it has yet to achieve the level of acceptance it has long held in Europe and the Pacific Rim countries. Chiropractic education, today, is on an equal quality and intensiveness level with medical and osteopathic education, in certain bio-mechanic, pharmacological and nutritional concentration areas, it is in fact advanced. This is definitely the case for business education, where Logan is in the lead not just in Chiropractic education, but in all health-care education. Logan graduates have been exposed to more business thoughts, concepts, and procedures then any other physicians at graduation.

The last complete study to develop a financial profile of chiropractors in the United States was done by the American Chiropractic Association in 1985. It is the feeling of the advisors to the practice that this information is now outdated. Therefore, the following information was developed by the advisors from their own client files of Franklin area offices. A "typical" Franklin chiropractor will need three to four years to develop the practice to a mature state. This is partially the result of the third-party reimbursement and payment factors in the industry. Delays of payment for fees of six to eight weeks are common, while "fee cutting" is becoming an occasional factor. These factors are being aggravated by "managed care" organizations such as HMOs and PPOs, an increasing factor in the health-care industry. While those organizations have not yet focused on the Chiropractors, it appears to be only a matter of time before they do. Additional delays can be expected if a patient's case involves litigation, as will occur in some worker's compensation and many accidental bodily injury situations. The "average" Franklin chiropractor can expect to generate approximately $150,000–$400,000 in annual fees per physician, on approximately two hundred to three hundred patient office visits per month. While both of these statistics are below those of medical and osteopathic physicians in the Franklin area, the "gap" has been closing over the last decade. A 92–95 percent collection ratio is common. On a cash accounting basis, overhead can be expected to run in the 30–40 percent range, depending mostly on the size and location of the office and the physician's and the effective and efficient use of staff. Common after-tax income to the Chiropractor is in the $60,000–$150,000 range for a physician in a mature practice.

Business Format and Responsibilities of the Principals

Freeman Chiropractic, P. C. will be an Indiana corporation with a charter issued under the Professional Corporation laws. Dr. Freeman will hold all outstanding share of the corporation and will serve as president and treasurer of the corporation, Mrs. Margaret (Peg) Freeman will serve as secretary.

Cash-flow Projections

As in all business startup situations, cash flow is crucial for survival and must, therefore, be tightly controlled. The principal and advisors are aware of the largely arbitrary value of "best estimate" forecasts and the high uncertainty factor involved in projections. Borrowing from the capital budgeting techniques, sensitivity analysis was used. Cash-flow projections were developed.

For the calendar year 1996, cash inflow projections were calculated on a weekly basis. Factors used in the projection of revenue (cash basis) are: new patients attracted to the practice, standard treatment protocol, standard office visit fee schedule, assumed patient mix (10 percent cash, 50 percent health insurance, 20 percent personal injury and litigated worker's comp, and 15 percent other), average third-party payment delay (eight weeks). In addition, projected visits and revenues from the established patients of Dr. Seller were included. These cash inflows are then recapitulated on a monthly basis to be merged with the cash outflow projections. Thus cash deficits can be projected on a monthly basis. The projection is attached at the end of this document. Details of all calculations are available upon request.

While these initial projections have a high degree of risk attached to them, it is the intent of the principals and advisors to update them on a regular basis (bimonthly) as experience is gained with actual operations. In this manner, it is anticipated that cash-flow control will become a tool used to assure survival, which in the first three years of operation equates to success. Risk is reduced as a result of the existing patient base and the resultant cash flow projected (conservatively). Approximately three hundred office visits per month from Dr. Seller's patients are included in the forecast.

Pro Forma Balance Sheets

The pro forma balance sheets, as shown in the financial statement section of the appendix, are presented in the format of generally accepted accounting procedures. Because of this, a few items must be noted to translate the statements to the real-world situation.

Cash in bank has been used as a balancing account other than in the opening balance sheet. Operating financial policy will be to keep a minimal balance in a corporate checking account and to maintain the remainder in a money-market type of fund. Of course, negotiation with a financial institution for the required loans may alter this plan. Inventory will consist of small quantities of orthopedic supports and implements together with nutritional supplements and vitamins for sale to patients. Accounts receivable will be mainly from third-party payors. Normal operating experience in the Franklin area indicates a forty-five to sixty days to cash period.

Furniture and equipment values indicate the value of both office and clinic equipment to be acquired in the process of acquisition of Dr. Seller's practice assets. A complete detailed list is available on request. Depreciation is calculated based on election of $17,500 expensing (section 179) in calendar year one and depreciation using the five year (half year convention) MACRS table.

Security deposits show a return of the deposits from the utility companies during the second full year of operation, and are to be acquired from the Seller practice. The real-estate deposit is expected to remain for the full seventy-two months of the lease. Organization expenses are being written off over the statutory seven years.

Taxes payable indicate an arbitrary amount owed for payroll taxes on December 31 of each year.

Equipment notes or leases show a pay off over sixty months with a moratorium or "contract payment" token amount during three or six months. Detailed amortization schedules are available upon request.

For certain tax and future financial flexibility purposes, legal capitalization has been kept to an absolute minimum. It is anticipated that income tax returns will be prepared on a cash accounting basis, rather then an accrual basis. Dr. Freeman may elect not to receive a salary during the first year to year and a half of operations should cash flow in the corporation require it. The main effect of this will be to reduce payroll and personal income taxes payable

Milestones and Critical Factors

As indicated earlier in this paper, opening day of the practice is anticipated to be April 15, 1996. A real-estate lease has been signed, the lease deposit will be taken over from Dr. Seller. The lease is a three-year lease with a three-year option to renew. It is effective April 15, 1996. The existing office facilities of Seller Chiropractic 4515 Main are well appointed and well suited for a chiropractic office. For the last eight years, Dr. Sellers has made continuous improvements to the leased space. It is a clean, bright, comfortable environment promoting positive, healthy attitudes.

Health care in the United States is in a state of change. State and national health-care proposals are being considered in the legislatures. Predicting the outcome of these deliberations is impossible at this stage, however, it appears that chiropractic will remain a viable health-care profession. With or without changes in law, third-party reimbursement rules and procedures will change in the next few years. While some of the changes may negatively influence the cash-flow position of health-care providers, they are not expected to endanger the success of this endeavor materially. Dr. Freeman feels poised to take advantage of changes which will open up positions for chiropractors in managed care networks. Two big Indiana managed care providers have accepted his applications and are currently in the process of credentialling the office.

Financing Proposal

Request is hereby made to arrange the debt financing required for the successful launch of the practice. Two alternatives are suggested:

A. Bank financing for the complete package as follows:
   1. A five-year term loan for the acquisition of the required equipment in the amount of approximately twenty-five thousand dollars.
   2. Establishing a working capital line of credit of no more than twenty thousand dollars, available for drawing until April 30, 1997.
   3. At that time, the principal anticipates combining the two loans into one note with a fixed or variable interest rate and a three- to five-year amortization schedule.
   4. Collateral offered are the equipment and furniture to be acquired, assignment of the accounts receivable, collateral assignment of adequate life and disability income policies on each of the two principals.
   5. Establishment of a long-term banking relationship for business and personal transactions of Dr. Freeman.

B. Bank financing for working capital only as follows:
   1. Establishing a working capital line of credit of no more than twenty thousand dollars, available for drawing until April 30, 1997.

2. At that time, the principals anticipate changing to a note with a fixed or variable interest rate and a three- to five-year amortization schedule.

3. Collateral offered are assignment of the accounts receivable, collateral assignment of adequate life and disability income policies on each of the two principals.

4 Establishment of a long-term banking relationship for business and personal transactions of Dr. Freeman.

Cash-Flow Projections
Freeman Chiropractic, P.C.

	1996 (10 months)	1997	1998
New Patient Office Visits (55,75,85)	495	675	765
Established Patient Office Visit	3,000	3,700	3,885
Total Office Visits	3,495	4,375	4,650
Beginning Cash from Operations	$0	$2,786	$5,860
Total Fees	$181,740	$227,500	$241,800
Total Collections	**$163,566**	**$204,750**	**$217,620**
Staff Salaries & PRT	$15,000	$18,900	$19,845
Rent	$14,280	$17,136	$17,136
Utilities	$1,750	$2,220	$2,331
Phone	$1,250	$1,500	$1,725
Supplies	$2,700	$3,500	$4,025
Dues & Subscriptions	$850	$1,075	$1,129
Advertising Expense	$5,000	$2,500	$2,000
Equipment Note Payment	$5,817	$6,981	$6,981
Repair & Maintenance	$1,500	$1,800	$1,980
Malpractice Insurance	$1,200	$1,600	$2,000
General Insurances	$1,800	$2,200	$2,200
Legal & Accounting	$1,500	$1,800	$1,800
Taxes & Licenses	$625	$900	$900
Seminars & Education	$1,500	$2,400	$3,600
Laundry & Uniforms	$550	$675	$725
Bank Expense	$400	$425	$475
Miscellaneous	$6,048	$7,007	$7,351
Working Capital Loan Payments	$583	$5,750	$0
Dr. Salaries & PRT	$30,000	$60,000	$100,000
Total Expenses	$92,353	$138,368	$176,202
Debt Service (Dr. Seller)	$65,426	$30,713	$3,861
Capital Acquisitions	$3,000	$3,311	$10,000
Corporate Income Tax Payments	$0	$29,284	$29,585
Net Annual Cash Flow	$2,786	$3,074	($2,029)
Cummulative Cash Flow from Operations	$2,786	$5,860	$3,831

Pro Forma Income Statements
Freeman Chiropractic PC

	1996	1997	1998
Total Collections	$163,566	$204,750	$217,620
Staff Salaries & PRT	$15,000	$18,900	$19,845
Rent	$14,280	$17,136	$17,136
Utilities	$1,750	$2,220	$2,331
Phone	$1,250	$1,500	$1,725
Supplies	$2,700	$3,500	$4,025
Dues & Subscriptions	$850	$1,075	$1,129
Advertising Expense	$5,000	$2,500	$2,000
Interest	$3,343	$3,561	$2,188
Repair & Maintenance	$1,500	$1,800	$1,980
Malpractice Insurance	$1,200	$1,600	$2,000
General Insurance	$1,800	$2,200	$2,200
Legal & Accounting	$1,500	$1,800	$1,800
Taxes & Licenses	$625	$900	$900
Seminars & Education	$1,500	$2,400	$3,600
Laundry & Uniforms	$550	$675	$725
Bank Expense	$400	$425	$475
Miscellaneous	$6,048	$7,007	$7,351
Depreciation, Expensing & Amortization	$25,052	$13,814	$19,143
Dr. Salaries & PRT	$30,000	$60,000	$100,000
Total Expenses	$114,349	$143,013	$190,553
Taxable Income	$49,217	$61,737	$27,067
Federal Income Tax	$13,781	$20,373	$7,579
State Income Tax (6%)	$2,953	$3,704	$1,624
Total Income Tax Payable	$16,734	$24,078	$9,203

Pro Forma Balance Sheets
Freeman Chiropractic PC

	Opening March 1996	Year End 1996	Year End 1997	1998
Assets				
Current Assets				
Cash in Bank	$3,350	$1,000	$1,250	$1,500
Inventory	$250	$250	$250	$250
Accounts Receivable	$0	$13,630	$17,060	$18,135
Total Current Assets	$3,600	$14,880	$18,560	$19,885
Fixed Assets				
Furniture & Equipment	$25,000	$28,000	$31,311	$41,311
Leasehold Improvements	$0	$0	$0	$0
Fixed Assets at Cost	$25,000	$28,000	$31,311	$41,311
Accumulated Depreciation	$0	$19,100	$25,771	$37,771
Net Fixed Assets	$25,000	$8,900	$5,540	$3,540
Other Assets				
Security Deposits	$1,400	$1,400	$1,100	$1,100
Patient Files Purchased	$50,000	$44,048	$36,905	$29,762
Organization Expenses	$1,000	$857	$714	$571
Total Other Assets	$52,400	$46,305	$38,719	$31,433
Total Assets	$81,000	$70,085	$62,819	$54,858
Liabilities and Equity				
Liabilities				
Current Liabilities				
Accounts Payable	$0	$0	$0	$0
Taxes Payable	$0	$300	$500	$700
Total Current Liabilities	$0	$300	$500	$700
Long-Term Liabilities				
Equipment Note	$25,000	$21,943	$17,773	$12,981
Working Capital Bank Note	$5,000	$0	$0	$0
Note Dr. Seller	$50,000	$44,048	$36,905	$29,762
Total Long-Term Liabilities	$80,000	$65,991	$54,678	$42,743
Total Liabilities	$80,000	$66,591	$55,678	$44,143
Equity				
Common Stock @ $1 par	$200	$200	$200	$200
Paid in Capital	$800	$800	$800	$800
Retained Earnings	$0	$2,794	$6,641	$10,415
Total Equity	$1.000	$3,794	$7,641	$11,415
Total Liabilities and Equity	$82,000	$74,179	$70,960	$66,973

Appendix I
If You Want To Know More—Resources

The authors feel an invaluable tool for any business owner is a resource list. Following are books, articles, and software recommendations the authors have found to be beneficial. Depending on your current need, be it foundation development, maintenance, or growth, there will be a resource for you to tap into.

Practice Motivation

Esteb, William D. *A Patient's Point of View.* Colorado Springs, Colorado: Orion Associates, Inc., 1995.

Esteb, William D. *Beyond Results.* Colorado Springs, Colorado: Orion Associates, Inc., 1995.

Esteb, William D. *Chiropractic Patientology.* Colorado Springs, Colorado: Orion Associates, Inc., 1995.

Esteb, William D. *Making Change.* Colorado Springs, Colorado: Orion Associates, Inc., 1995.

Esteb, William D. *My Report of Findings.* Colorado Springs, Colorado: Orion Associates, Inc., 1995.

Joseph, Vince, and Cox Joseph, Terri. *Adjustments.* Norfolk, Virginia: Hampton Roads Publishing Company, Inc., 1993.

National Board of Chiropractic Examiners, *Job Analysis of Chiropractic,* a project report, survey analysis, and summary of the practice of chiropractic within the United States, (NBCE, 1993). 901-54th Avenue, Greeley, CO. Phone (303)356-9100.

Business Conceptual Development

Adizes, Ichak. *Corporate Life Cycles: how and why corporations grow and die and what to do about it.* Englewood Cliffs, New Jersey: Prentice-Hall, Inc., 1988.

Drucker, Peter F. *The New Realities: in government and politics/ in economics and business/ in society and world view.* New York: Truman Talley Books/Dutton, 1990.

Kuratko, Donald, and Hodgett, Richard. *Entrepreneurship, a contemporary approach.* Orlando, Florida: Harcourt Brace, 1992.

Naisbitt, John. *Megatrends: ten new directions transforming our lives.* New York: Morrow, 1990.

Peters, Tom. *Thriving on Chaos: a handbook for a management revolution.* New York: Random House, 1987.

Senge, Peter M. *The Fifth Discipline: the art & practice of the learning organization.* New York: Currency, 1990.

Business Practice Needs
Computer

Dummy Books (computers, business, forms) IDG Books.

Internet sources.

Medisoft Patient Accounting Software. Mesa, Arizona. Phone (800)333-4747.

Typing and/or computer programs and skills (keyboarding, word processing, spreadsheets) Check with local community colleges

Marketing

Sachs, Laura. *Do-it-Yourself Marketing for the Professional Practice.* Englewood Cliffs, New Jersey: Prentice-Hall, Inc., 1986. (This book is out of print; if you find one, grab it. This book is well worth the $40–$80 it will cost.)

Insurance

Fordney, Marilyn. *The Insurance Handbook for the Medical Office*(forms). Philadelphia: Sanders, 1995.

McAndrews, Jerome F., D.C. *Managed Care: a guide for new practitioners.* West Des Moines, Iowa: National Chiropractic Mutual Insurance Company, 1996.

Forms

Back Talk Systems, Inc., 2845 Ore Mill Drive, Suite 4, Colorado Springs, CO, 80904-3161. Phone (800) 937-3113.

Patient Education Material

Back Talk Systems, Inc. (Super information: video tapes, wall posters, pamphlets, report of findings and consultations, flip charts—all designed from the patient point of view.) 2845 Ore Mill Drive, Suite 4, Colorado Springs, CO, 80904-3161. Phone (800) 937-3113.

Personal motivation

Covey, Stephen R. *The 7 Habits of Highly Effective People.* New York: Simon & Schuster, Inc., 1989.

Sinetar, Marsha. *Do What You Love, The Money Will Follow.* New York: Dell Publishing, 1987.

Risk Management

National Chiropractic Mutual Insurance Company, 1452 29th Street, Suite 102, West Des Moines, Iowa, 50266-1307. Phone (800) 247-8043.

Professional Organizations

International Chiropractic Association, 1110 North Glede Rd., Arlington, VA 22201.

American Chiropractic Association, 1701 Clarendon Blvd., Arlington, VA 22209.

Bibliography

Books

Brown, H. *Life's Little Instruction Book.* Nashville, Tennessee: Rutledge Hill Press, 1991.

Elliott, D. *Ethics of Asking: Dilemma in Higher Education Fundraising.* Baltimore, Maryland: The Johns Hopkins University Press, 1995.

Fisher, J. *Power of the Presidency.* New York, New York: Collier MacMillian Publishers, 1984.

Morris, Robert, *Robert Morris Associates Annual Statement Studies.* Philadelphia: Robert Morris Associates, 1996.

Penick, H. *The Game for a Lifetime,* New York, New York: Simon and Schuster, 1996.

Pezzullo, T. and Brittingham, P. *Fund Raising in Higher Education: Ethical Questions.* (ASHE-ERIC Higher Education Report No. 1). Washington, D.C.: The George Washington University, 1990.

Rosofsky, H. The University: *An Owner's Manual.* New York, New York: W.W. Norton and Company, 1990.

Standard and Poor's Industry Surveys, New York: McGraw-Hill, 1997.

Brochures or Phamplets

Guide to Preemployment Inquiries. Des Moines, Iowa: Job Service of Iowa, 1994.

Federal Employer's Tax Guide (Circular E), Washington, D.C.: Internal Revenue Service, 1997.

Periodicals

Rubinstein, Carin, *Psychology Today,* "Wellness is All," October 1982.

National Research Corporation health survey, *Modern Health Care,* April 1985.

Index

Index of Figures

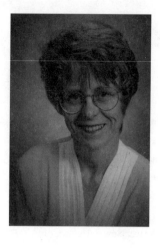

Gayle A. Jensen is the president and founder of Practice Consultants, Inc., an Iowa-based firm addressing the development and maintenance needs of new and experienced chiropractic physicians, and coordinating medical cases for attorneys and their clients.

She has earned graduate credit at St. Ambrose University in business administration and has her bachelor of science degree in nursing from the University of Iowa. Gayle has conducted seminars on topics covering practice development and court and deposition testimony preparation. She has been a guest lecturer at Logan College of Chiropractic, Palmer College of Chiropractic, and Cleveland Chiropractic College of Kansas City.

Gayle has worked in many roles, from clinic nurse, receptionist, and office manager, to clinical coordinator of a multidoctor chiropractic clinic. These varied roles have given Gayle a unique perspective and a set of experiences that she shares with the profession.

Rudolf P. Vrugtman is a full-time instructor at Logan College of Chiropractic. He developed and has taught business administration courses for the last fifteen years. In addition to his teaching responsibility, he is a consultant to the Health Center Chief of Staff on business matters. Rudi teaches on a part-time basis at the College of Business and Management, St. Louis Academic Center, National Louis University.

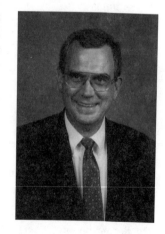

After owning a consulting firm for over twenty years and working with many small business owners in starting and operating their ventures, Rudi accepted an invitation to become a full-time instructor in 1995. He continues to maintain contact with large numbers of chiropractors throughout the country and assists new practices during their startup phase. He is enrolled in graduate school and expects to receive his Ph.D. in the summer of 1999.